MW01600334

Omega-3 Fatty Acids in Health and Disease

FOOD SCIENCE AND TECHNOLOGY

A Series of Monographs, Textbooks, and Reference Books

1. Flavor Research: Principles and Techniques, *R. Teranishi, I. Hornstein, P. Issenberg, and E. L. Wick (out of print)*
2. Principles of Enzymology for the Food Sciences, *John R. Whitaker*
3. Low-Temperature Preservation of Foods and Living Matter, *Owen R. Fennema, William D. Powrie, and Elmer H. Marth*
4. Principles of Food Science
   Part I: Food Chemistry, *edited by Owen R. Fennema*
   Part II: Physical Methods of Food Preservation, *Marcus Karel, Owen R. Fennema, and Daryl B. Lund*
5. Food Emulsions, *edited by Stig Friberg*
6. Nutritional and Safety Aspects of Food Processing, *edited by Steven R. Tannenbaum*
7. Flavor Research: Recent Advances, *edited by R. Teranishi, Robert A. Flath, and Hiroshi Sugisawa*
8. Computer-Aided Techniques in Food Technology, *edited by Israel Saguy*
9. Handbook of Tropical Foods, *edited by Harvey T. Chan*
10. Antimicrobials in Foods, *edited by Alfred Larry Branen and P. Michael Davidson*
11. Food Constituents and Food Residues: Their Chromatographic Determination, *edited by James F. Lawrence*
12. Aspartame: Physiology and Biochemistry, *edited by Lewis D. Stegink and L. J. Filer, Jr.*
13. Handbook of Vitamins: Nutritional, Biochemical, and Clinical Aspects, *edited by Lawrence J. Machlin*
14. Starch Conversion Technology, *edited by G. M. A. van Beynum and J. A. Roels*

Food Processing Operations and Scale-up, *Kenneth J. Valentas, Leon Levine, and J. Peter Clark*

Handbook of Vitamins, Second Edition, Revised and Expanded, *edited by Lawrence J. Machlin*

Omega-3 Fatty Acids in Health and Disease

edited by

Robert S. Lees

*Harvard University and Massachusetts Institute of Technology
and New England Deaconess Hospital
Boston, Massachusetts*

Marcus Karel

*Massachusetts Institute of Technology
Cambridge, Massachusetts*

MARCEL DEKKER, INC.   **New York and Basel**

Library of Congress Cataloging-in-Publication Data

Omega-3 fatty acids in health and disease.

(Food science and technology ; 37)
1. Omega-3 fatty acids.   2. Fish oil in human nutrition.
    I. Lees, Robert S.   II. Karel, Marcus.
III. Title: Omega-three fatty acids in health and disease.
IV. Series: Food science and technology (Marcel Dekker); 37.
QP752.044044 1990   612.3'97   89-25877
ISBN 0-8247-8292-5 (alk. paper)

This report describes the results of research performed as part of
the MIT Sea Grant College Program MITSG89-2 with support
from the Office of Sea Grant in the National Oceanic and Atmos-
pheric Administration, Department of Commerce, through Grant
No. NA86AA-D-SG089 and from the Massachusetts Institute of
Technology.

This book is printed on acid-free paper.

MARCEL DEKKER, INC.
270 Madison Avenue, New York, New York 10016

Current printing (last digit):
10 9 8 7 6 5 4 3 2 1

PRINTED IN THE UNITED STATES OF AMERICA

Preface

Fish has become big business. Not only is the consumption of fish by the American public almost 50% higher than it was two decades ago, but a whole new industry has arisen: the refining and marketing of fish oils as a pharmaceutical product, generally in the form of capsules for dietary supplementation. This upsurge of interest has occurred because an increasing body of data suggests that fish and fish oil have beneficial effects on human health. These effects—a reduction in symptoms and death from cardiovascular disease, arthritis, and cancer, according to the proponents of fish oil—are thought to be caused by certain fish oil fatty acids that are chemically different from those in other human foods. These fatty acids, called omega-3 ("ω-3" or "n-3") fatty acids, are polyunsaturated, but the double bonds are in different locations in the molecule than those in the more familiar plant fatty acids, such as linoleic and arachidonic acids.

This volume will discuss several major aspects of the relationship between fish oil and human health. The first part of this book will deal with the effects of dietary fats on human health, citing and weighing the evidence that fish or fish oil consumption affects the incidence of hypertension and coronary heart disease, rheumatic diseases, and cancer. The effects of dietary omega-3 fatty acids on blood lipids and on platelet activity will be reviewed in detail. The epidemiologic evidence concerning the consumption of fish and human health will be evaluated, and the implications for medical care and public health policy will be explored.

The second part of the book is concerned with the science, technology, economics, and legal aspects of the delivery of omega-3 fatty acids to the consuming public. It will address the sources of these fatty acids and the strategies for their utilization for optimal nutrition. The availability of these lipids within traditional dietary sources, as well as the utilization of nutritional supplements, will be reviewed. The methods for producing fish oil, the problems with standardization and preservation of the relatively unstable omega-3 fatty acids, and the regulatory aspects of fish oil as a food and a drug will be considered.

The editors hope that this will provide needed information for the clinician, medical research scientist, food scientist, and epidemiologist, and also for the businessman concerned with the marine fishery industry and the layman concerned with nutrition. We hope, as well, that this volume will point up the gaps in our knowledge, and focus attention on additional studies that need to be carried out in order to promote rational use of fish and fish oils.

Robert S. Lees
Marcus Karel

Contents

Contributors

Robert G. Ackman, B.A., M.Sc., Ph.D., DIC   Canadian Institute of Fisheries Technology, Technical University of Nova Scotia, Halifax, Nova Scotia, Canada

Julie E. Buring, D.Sc.   Department of Preventive Medicine, Harvard Medical School and Brigham and Women's Hospital, Boston, Massachusetts

Kenneth K. Carroll, B.Sc., M.Sc., M.A., Ph.D.   Department of Biochemistry, University of Western Ontario, London, Ontario, Canada

Charles H. Hennekens, M.D.   Departments of Medicine and Preventive Medicine, Harvard Medical School and Brigham and Women's Hospital, Boston, Massachusetts

D. Roger Illingworth, M.D., Ph.D.   Division of Endocrinology, Metabolism and Clinical Nutrition, Department of Medicine, Oregon Health Sciences University, Portland, Oregon

John E. Kinsella, Ph.D. Department of Food Biochemistry, Institute of Food Science, Cornell University, Ithaca, New York

Val Krukonis Phasex Corporation, Lawrence, Massachusetts

Robert S. Lees, M.D. Division of Health Sciences and Technology, Harvard University and Massachusetts Institute of Technology, and New England Deaconess Hospital, Boston, Massachusetts

Sherry L. Mayrent, Ph.D. Department of Medicine, Harvard Medical School and Brigham and Women's Hospital, Boston, Massachusetts

Richard J. Radmer, Ph.D. Martek Corporation, Columbia, Maryland

W. M. N. Ratnayake, Ph.D.* Canadian Institute of Fisheries Technology, Technical University of Nova Scotia, Halifax, Nova Scotia, Canada

Artemis P. Simopoulos, M.D.† Division of Nutritional Sciences, International Life Sciences Institute of Research Foundation, Washington, D.C.

Roy Soberman, M.D. Department of Rheumatology and Immunology, Brigham and Women's Hospital, Boston, Massachusetts

Daniel Ullmann, D.Sc.(Med), M.P.H. Division of Endocrinology, Metabolism and Clinical Nutrition, Department of Medicine, Oregon Health Sciences University, Portland, Oregon

Current affiliations:
*Food Directorate, Health and Welfare Canada, Ottawa, Ontario, Canada
†The Center for Genetics, Nutrition and Health, American Association for World Health, Washington, D.C.

Part I: Health Effects of Omega-3 Fatty Acids

1
Impact of Dietary Fat on Human Health

Robert S. Lees
Harvard University and Massachusetts Institute of Technology
and New England Deaconess Hospital
Boston, Massachusetts

INTRODUCTION

Human beings, for many centuries, have attributed almost mystical properties to their dietary fats. The ancient Romans not only ate their beloved olive oil, they anointed themselves with it. Modern Americans not only eat fish in hope that its oil will keep them healthy, they swallow fish oil capsules as a drug. In this discussion, I will attempt to review the salient facts concerning dietary fat and its effects on human health. My goal is to provide an overview, since the details of each of the major categories of disease with which dietary fats have been associated will be given by others later in this volume.

To my mind, the modern era of dietary fat research began with an animal, rather than a human experiment. Parenthetically, I will cite relatively few animal data here, because laboratory animal experiments are often not extrapolable to the situation in the free-living human being. The experiment I have in mind, however, is highly extrapolable. In the early 1920s, Simon Henry Gage and Pierre Fish, at Cornell University, fed a sheep some vegetable oil colored with a fat-soluble dye called cochineal. Then they dissected the sheep and found that the animal's intestinal lymph, or chyle, contained tiny droplets of fat which contained the dye, and that these droplets passed into the blood via the thoracic lymph duct. Finally, after several hours, the sheep's fat turned pink. In a preliminary publication (Gage, 1920) in *Cornell Veterinarian*, Gage named these small particles "chylomicrons," the name we use today. In a later full publication (Gage and Fish, 1924), the investigators postulated that the function of chylomicrons was to transport dietary fat into the lymph and from there to the bloodstream and sites of storage or utilization, the function that they are still thought to fulfill. This classic experiment in fat metabolism is, to my knowledge, the first metabolic experiment to use a tracer. The studies of Gage and Fish, which graphically showed the passage of dietary fat through the lymph and blood to the depot fat, set the stage for the next half-century of studies on the metabolism of dietary fat and its effects on human health.

In the spirit of Gage and Fish, we must turn to the composition and the metabolism of dietary fat in order to understand its effects on health. What we eat (Table 1) contains three major lipid classes, triglycerides, phospholipids, and sterols, plus a number of minor components of varying, sometimes major, importance. This list, which is by no means comprehensive, gives us some idea of both the variety and the variability of human dietary fat intake. Commercial vegetable oils, for instance, may contain almost pure triglycerides, the sterols and phospholipids having been removed to ensure clarity. Egg yolk, by contrast, is about 65% triglycerides, 25% phopholipids, and 5% cholesterol. When discussing human disease, one must distinguish among substrate effects, the effects of natural minor components of metabolic importance, and the effects of toxic minor components. Let us turn at this point to normal human fat metabolism.

Table 1 Some Components of Human Dietary Fats

Component	Subclasses	Natural/otherwise	Percent of total
Triglycerides	Saturated	Natural/synthetic	65-95+
	Monounsaturated	Natural/synthetic	
	Polyunsaturated	Natural	
Phospholipids	Lecithins	Natural/synthetic	1-30
	Other phosphatides	Natural	
Sterols	Cholesterol	Natural	0-5
	Other animal sterols	Natural	
	Plant sterols	Natural	
Vitamins and	Retinol	Natural/synthetic	
provitamins	Caroteins	Natural	<1%
	Vitamin D	Synthetic	
	Tocopherols	Natural/synthetic	
Hydrocarbons	Squalene	Natural	<1%
	Alkanes, alkenes		
	Polycyclics	Environmental contaminants	
Antioxidants	BHA/BHT	Added to prolong shelf life	<1%
	Propyl gallate		
	Tocopherols		
Environmental toxins	DDT	Insecticide	
	PCBs	Insulating fluid	<<1%
	Mycotoxins	Food spoilage	
	Other toxins		
Other additives	Silicones	Nonstick agents	<<1%

HUMAN FAT METABOLISM

Fat fulfills multiple functions in the human body, acting as the major metabolic fuel to meet caloric needs, as the major structural component of the cell wall, and as an essential precursor of several hormones critical to normal existence. A complete review of human fat metabolism is beyond the scope of this chapter and this volume; the interested reader is encouraged to seek out other, excellent, sources of this information (Lewis, 1976; Havel et al., 1980, Assmann, 1982). However, the major pathways of fat metabolism will be discussed here, as they are essential to understanding the topics that follow.

Of the three major lipid classes in dietary fat, sterols have the simplest metabolic pathway in most respects, and triglycerides the most complex. Nevertheless, we will begin with the latter, as it is necessary to understand triglyceride metabolism in order to place that of the other lipids into proper perspective. The majority of dietary fat is triglycerides, which pass through the stomach unaltered by its acid pH and the gastric proteases. In the small intestine (Fig. 1), the pH is alkaline, and the pancreatic juice that is secreted into the small intestine contains a powerful lipase (Semeriva and Desnuelle, 1979), which with its polypeptide colipase (Borgstrom, 1979) has the ability to hydrolyze triglycerides to monoglycerides and 2 moles per mole of free fatty acids (FFA). Pancreatic lipase is virtually inactive on triglycerides in their usual bulk state, however. The enzyme's activity depends on the emulsification of dietary fat into micelles, small spheres of triglycerides, along with any other nonpolar lipids present in the dietary fat, such as sterol esters and fat-soluble vitamins, with a surface coat of phospholipids, free cholesterol, and bile acids. Most of the first two and all of the third of these polar lipids of the micellar surface come from the bile, which is secreted by the liver, with intermediate storage in the gallbladder and bile ducts. Bile is secreted into the small intestine when fat enters it from the stomach. This process (Fig. 1) is triggered by the hormone cholecystokinin, which is secreted by the duodenal mucosa when fat comes into contact with it.

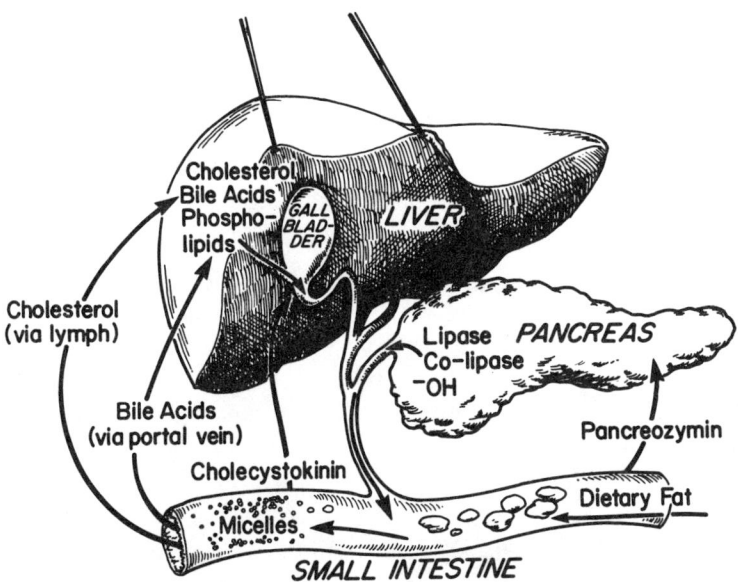

Figure 1 The mechanisms of fat digestion and absorption (see also Fig. 2). Dietary fat is solubilized by bile acids, phospholipids, and free cholesterol, all of which enter the gut from the gallbladder bile. It is then digested by pancreatic lipase which is secreted in the pancreatic juice. Bile acids are absorbed directly and retransported to the liver via the portal vein. Cholesterol and triglycerides are absorbed as chylomicrons; the cholesterol is returned to the liver via a circuitous route. See text for further details.

The monoglycerides and free fatty acids produced by lipase activity are absorbed by diffusion into the gut mucosal cells and there resynthesized into triglycerides, with the admixture of 10-20% of endogenous fatty acids (i.e., fatty acids from the body stores, not from the digested fat) and assembled into *chylomicrons*. The chylomicrons, as described by Gage and Fish, pass into the intestinal lymphatics, from there into the large lymphatic chamber in the abdomen called the cisternal chyli, and finally via

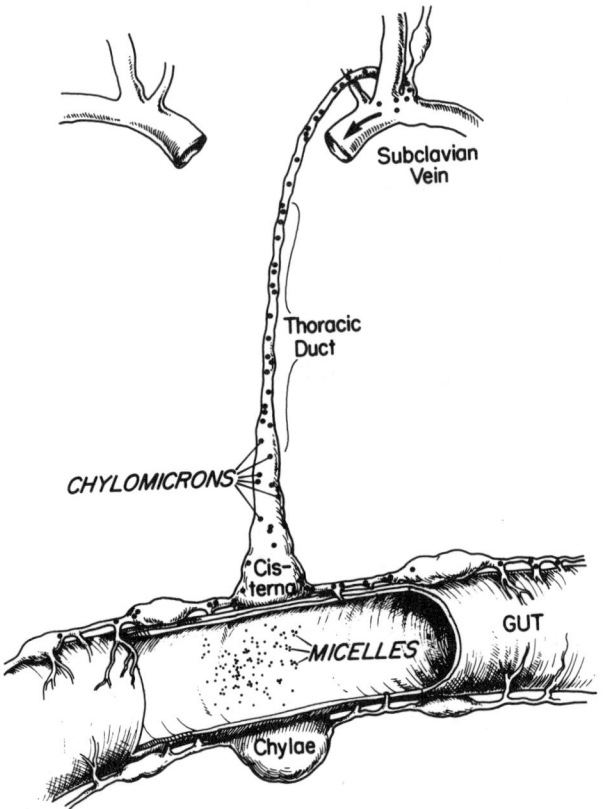

Figure 2 Chylomicron synthesis and transport. Both the dietary triglycerides and cholesterol are absorbed into the intestinal mucosal cells and incorporated into chylomicrons, which move from these cells sequentially into the intestinal lymph capillaries, the larger intestinal lymphatics, the thoracic lymph duct, and finally the venous blood by the route shown. See text for details.

the thoracic (lymphatic) duct into the venous blood (Fig. 2). The chylomicrons then pass through the heart in the venous blood, and chylomicrons are distributed to the entire body via the arterial and finally the capillary circulation. There, something akin to the mirror image of chylomicron production occurs. As the chylomicrons move along the capillary surface, their triglycerides are lipolyzed by the concerted action of two important enzymes—lipoprotein li-

pase (LPL) and lecithin:cholesterol acyl transferase (LCAT). LPL
and a related enzyme, hepatic lipase, hydrolyze the triglycerides
to glycerol and free fatty acids. The free fatty acids diffuse
through the capillaries into the underlying parenchymal cells,
where they are either burned as metabolic fuel or resynthesized
to triglycerides and stored. The glycerol is returned via the blood
to the liver, where it enters the hepatic glycerol pool and may be
resynthesized into triglycerides, converted to carbohydrate, or it
may undergo one of many other metabolic reactions. Since as
much as 100 g of dietary fat may be absorbed and transported
through the blood each day, the process of chylomicron formation
and transport must be swift and efficient. The half-life of chylomicrons in plasma, for example, is about 10 min in normal human
beings. Thus, the triglyceride fatty acids from dietary fat are rapidly and efficiently transported to peripheral tissues, where they
may be stored, as in the adipose tissue, or burned for energy as
occurs in muscle. Many metabolic studies (Fredrickson and Gordon, 1958, Fritz, 1961; Cahill et al., 1966) have shown that up to
50% in the fed state and up to 90% of the total fasting caloric
needs of human beings are met by the metabolism of fatty acids.

What, then, happens in the fasting state? How are metabolic
needs met when dietary fat is not directly supplying chylomicron
fatty acids? The human body has an alternative system for supplying fatty acids for metabolism (Fig. 3). Depot fat has a rich
sympathetic innervation and is vascularized with an extensive capillary network. Norepinephrine, delivered at the sympathetic
nerve endings, and circulating epinephrine and norepinephrine,
delivered via the capillary blood, activate a hormone-sensitive lipase in adipose tissue which rapidly lyses triglycerides into glycerol and FFA. These molecules rapidly move down a concentration gradient across the capillary endothelium into the blood. The
FFA bind immediately to the plasma albumin, which has many
high-affinity FFA binding sites (Goodman, 1958; Spector, 1975).
They are then transported via the blood to muscle, where they are
extracted and burned for energy.

Any unburned FFA are removed efficiently by the liver, as
is the glycerol, resynthesized into triglycerides, and resecreted as

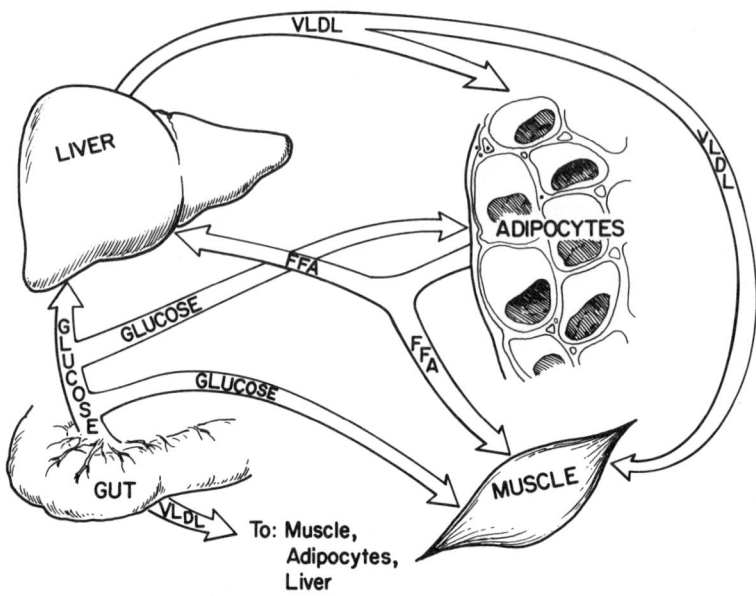

Figure 3 The interactions of glucose and fatty acid metabolism. Each of the multiple alternative pathways shown may change in its fractional contribution according to the metabolic state of the individual. The details of these complex interactions are summarized in the text.

triglyceride-rich very-low-density lipoproteins (VLDL, Fig. 3). When blood glucose is also low, the glycerol returned to the liver is converted to glucose, and the fatty acids to "ketone bodies" (the oxygenated fatty acids beta-hydroxybutyric and acetoacetic), which are alternative fuels for the brain in place of glucose. The neural and hormonal sympathetic control of fatty acid mobilization is so sensitive and rapid that significant rises in FFA concentration can be detected within a few seconds of a stimulus that disturbs a person—a loud noise, for instance, or a perceived physical threat. If the mobilized FFA are not burned for energy, they are reesterified by the liver and returned to the adipose stores as VLDL. The cycle of endogenous fatty acid availability is not only finely tuned, it is rapid, much like that for chylomicrons. The half-life of FFA in the blood is about 2 min and that of VLDL about 1 hr in normal subjects. As much as 100 g or more of fat may pass through this cycle each day.

Cholesterol metabolism, by contrast, is relatively indolent. In most human beings on a Western diet, cholesterol intake is between 0.5 and 1 g daily. It is consumed as a component of animal fat, almost always accompanied by a much larger amount of triglycerides. There is no cholesterol in vegetable fat—the critical biochemical distinction between plants and animals is that *only* animals can synthesize cholesterol. Dietary cholesterol, as noted above, is incorporated into micelles in the small intestine. It is almost all free cholesterol, so no hydrolytic step is necessary. From that point its fate is very different from that of triglycerides. First, it is diluted by a much larger amount of biliary cholesterol. Then, rather than being almost completely absorbed, as are triglycerides, it is only partially absorbed, and its percent absorption varies widely, depending both on how much cholesterol is in a given meal and on what other lipids are included in the meal (Quintao et al., 1971). In general, about 50-75% of dietary cholesterol is absorbed at low intakes, and this falls progressively to 25% or less at high dietary intakes (Borgstrom, 1969; Quintao et al., 1971). Once it reaches the gut mucosal cell, the cholesterol again behaves very differently from triglycerides. It enters the blood stream only very slowly, over a period of 24 hr or more after a given meal, and only in part as chylomicron cholesterol. Much of the dietary cholesterol is probably secreted into the portal venous blood as intestinally synthesized VLDL. At the same time, endogenous cholesterol synthesis goes on in virtually every cell in the body, although half or more of the total occurs in a single organ, the liver. Total endogenous synthesis is about 1 g/day, and in human beings, unlike many animals, changes relatively little as dietary intake changes. This important and underappreciated fact means that the more cholesterol a person eats, the more the body accumulates, despite its poor absorption (Bergstrom, 1969, Quintao et al., 1971).

Cholesterol can leave the human body by only a few restricted pathways. The most important is the gut. Much of the endogenously synthesized cholesterol in the liver is secreted into the bile either as such or as bile acids, an oxidative breakdown product of cholesterol. The bile eventually ends up in the intesttine, where much of the biliary cholesterol and most of the bile acids are reabsorbed and eventually returned to the liver (Carey, 1982, Hofmann et al., 1983, Hofmann, 1984). This enterohepatic circulation of cholesterol and bile acids is an important control mechanism for body sterol metabolism and is the site at which certain cholesterol-lowering drugs act, for instance. Some of the biliary cholesterol, some of the bile acids, and some of the dietary cholesterol—that which is not absorbed or reabsorbed—is excreted in the stools. Ideally, the total excreted would equal the sum of that consumed in the diet plus that syntheized, since the only other sources of cholesterol loss or catabolism are via the small amount of skin that is desquamated each day and the few milligrams of cholesterol that are converted into steroid hormones by the adrenals and the gonads. In reality, most human beings are in very slightly positive cholesterol balance and slowly deposit cholesterol over time in their adipose and connective tissues (Crouse et al., 1972) and, unfortunately for many, in the walls of their arteries.

The fate of dietary phospholipids is relatively simple. They are hydrolyzed almost quantitatively in the small intestine by pancreatic phospholipases and their multiple constituents absorbed and mixed in the gut metabolic pools of fatty acid, phosphoric acid, choline, and so on. Phospholipids can be synthesized and broken down by every nucleated cell in the body, so there is little need for net phospholipid transport. In terms of fat absorption, their major role is as a primary constituent of the bile and one of the two biliary detergents (the other being bile acids) that emulsify the dietary triglycerides and cholesterol into micelles and facilitate hydrolysis and absorption of the former and partial absorption of the latter.

As can be noted from Table 1, there are many other lipids, at least potentially, in human dietary fat. Several are important to consideration of the role of dietary fat in etiology of disease and will be mentioned briefly here. The reader is encouraged to consult the cited references for the details of their chemistry and metabolism. These other lipids include plant sterols (Tilvis and Miettinen, 1986), animal sterols other than cholesterol (Lin et al., 1984), fat-soluble vitamins (Machlin, 1984), antioxidants (Coppen, 1983, Liliger, 1983) and environmental toxins, both natural toxins such as mycotoxins (Wogan and Busby, 1980) and man-made toxins such as polychlorinated biphenyls (PCBs), insecticides such as DDT, and herbicides such as dioxins (McEwen and Stephenson, 1979; Poland and Knutson, 1982).

Plant and animal sterols are specifically important in the understanding of lipid-lipid interactions in the maintenance of plasma cholesterol concentrations and deserve review here. Plant sterols (Fig. 4) are found in all vegetable oils in their natural state, but are usually removed from the oils for the commercial marketplace. Their limited solubility in triglycerides often causes turbidity and precipitation on the shelf and thus decreases the eye appeal of the vegetable oil to the purchaser. These plant sterols, which generally differ from cholesterol in that they have side-chain aliphatic substituents (Fig. 4), are more poorly absorbed than cholesterol, except in certain rare inherited states (Bhattacharyya and Connor, 1974, Salen et al., 1985a,b), and themselves inhibit cholesterol absorption, presumably by blocking cholesterol-binding sites on the gut mucosal cells. Thus, their frequent removal from food fats is probably not beneficial from a public health point of view. Sterols like campesterol and beta-sitosterol are present in low concentration in normal human blood plasma (Gould et al., 1969, Salen et al., 1970; Lees and Lees, 1976, Gregg et al., 1986) and are occasionally found in tumors, presumably secondarily, but except in the rare subjects who lack the normal absorption barrier for them (Bhattacharyya and Connor, 1974; Gregg et al., 1986), they do not cause disease. Other plant sterols, such as ergosterol (Fig. 4), are vitamin D precursors (Machlin, 1984).

Not very many years ago, it was thought that clam and oyster sterols, like those of shrimp and lobster, were almost pure choles-

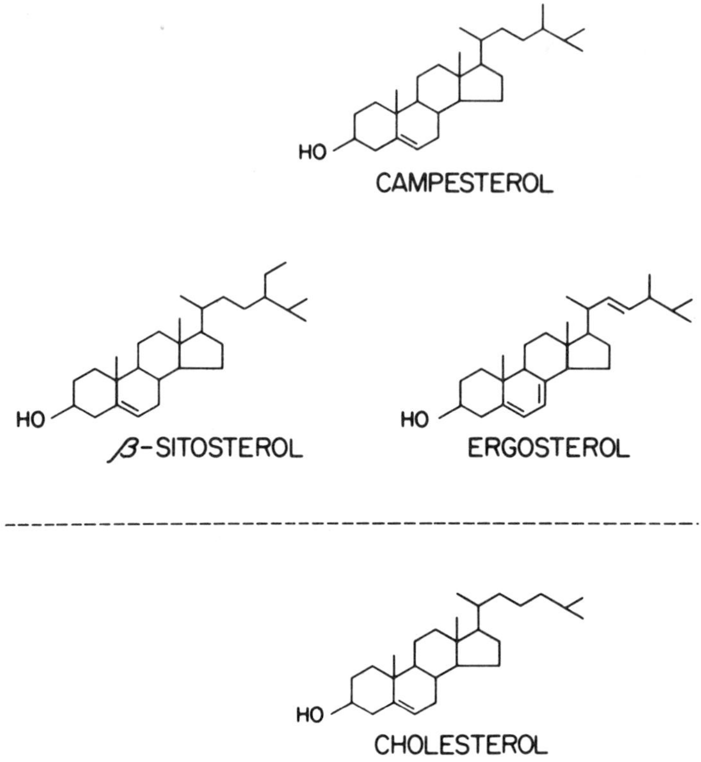

CAMPESTEROL

β-SITOSTEROL

ERGOSTEROL

CHOLESTEROL

Figure 4 Some common plant sterols. All differ in the side chain from cholesterol, shown for comparison below the dotted line. Ergosterol has, in addition to the side-chain methyl substituent, two double bonds not present in cholesterol.

terol. Recent research, mostly from the laboratory of Connor and his colleagues in Oregon (Connor and Lin, 1981), has shown that there is a marked difference between the sterols of the mollusks, i.e., oysters and clams, and those of crustaceans, such as shrimp, crayfish, and lobster. The latter have largely cholesterol, whereas mollusk sterols are only about 50% cholesterol and include several other compounds (Fig. 5), some of which, although clearly animal sterols, share with the plant sterols the property of poor absorbability. Others are well absorbed, however, and, like cholesterol, appear in both the bile and the blood (Connor and Lin, 1981,

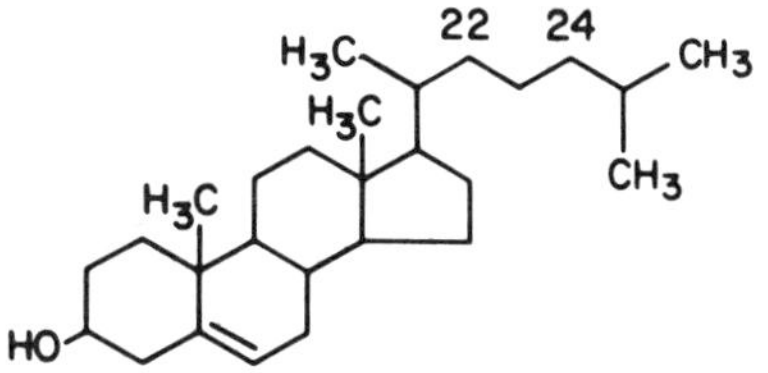

CHOLESTEROL

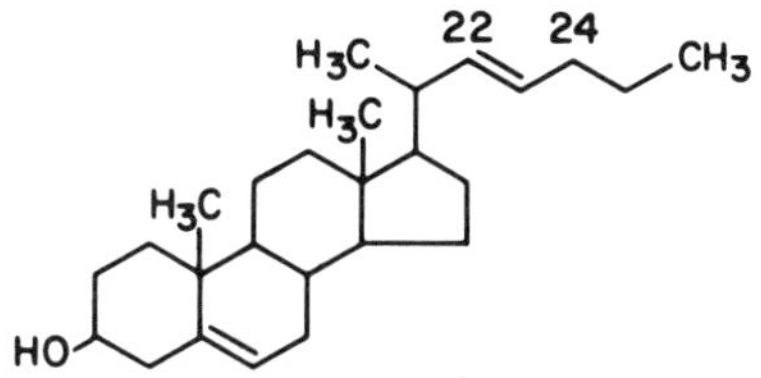

25-DESMETHYL
22-DEHYDRO-
CHOLESTEROL

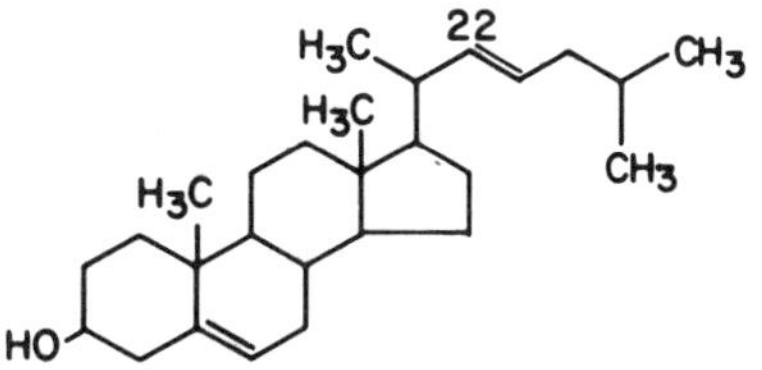

22-DEHYDRO-
CHOLESTEROL

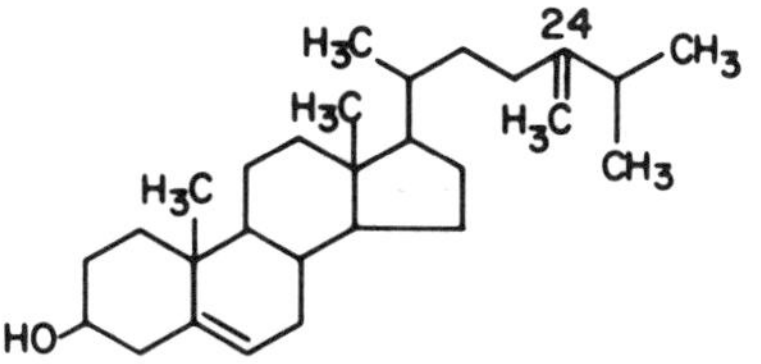

24-METHYLENE
CHOLESTEROL

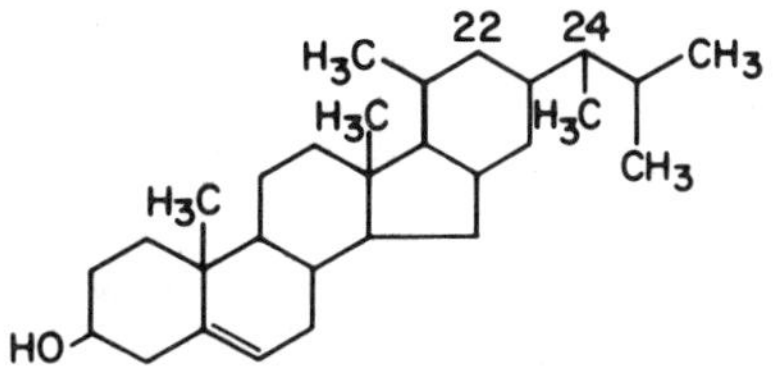

BRASSICASTEROL

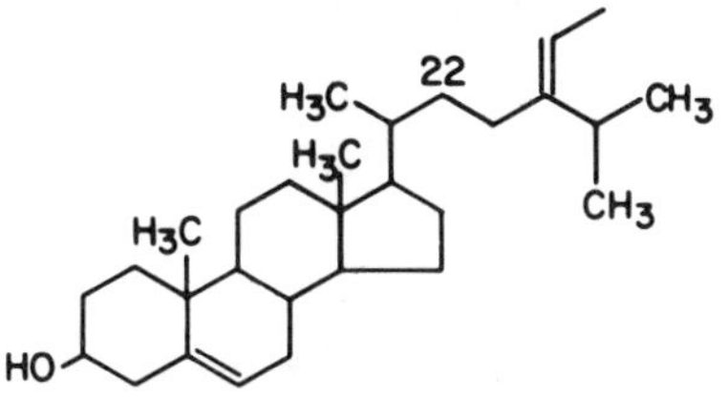

ISOFUCOSTEROL

Figure 5 The structure of a number of stererols found in mol-usks. Some of these are less well absorbed than cholesterol; see text for details.

1982). In limited clinical studies (Connor and Lin, 1982), crusta-cean ingestion was associated with a modest rise in plasma choles-terol while mollusk ingestion raised plasma cholesterol in a hyper-cholesterolemic patient, but not in six normal men.

An old and empirical observation in human fat metabolism, that certain polyunsaturated fatty acids must be in the diet in order for normal growth and sustained health to occur, has been elegantly explained by the biochemical findings that these acids are essential precursors of a whole series of highly active substances that have profound effects on smooth muscle cells throughout the body, including those in the vascular, uterine, and bronchial walls, as well as on blood platelets, to cause or inhibit aggregation. These hormones, called, as a class, eicosanoids, include prostaglandins, thromboxanes, leukotrienes, and lipoxins, and are produced by oxidation of certain polyunsaturated fatty acids (PUFA) that cannot be synthesized by mammals and must be obtained from plant sources (McGiff, 1980, Stenson and Parker, 1984, Samuelsson et al., 1987). The pathways of oxidative metabolism of PUFA are diagrammed in Figure 6, with arachidonic acid used as an example. Arachidonic acid is a representative of one of two naturally occurring series of polyunsaturated fatty acids (Fig. 7), which are metabolically equivalent and often interconvertible, but only within a given series. Furthermore, each series produces metabolically distinct oxidation products and these differences may have profound implications for disease, as will be discussed in detail in Chapters 2,4, and 6. The more common fatty acids, which are synthesized by many terrestrial plants, have the first of their two or more double bonds six carbon atoms in from the methyl end of the carbon chain and are therefore called "n-6" or "ω-6" fatty acids (Fig. 7). These include linoleic acid and arachidonic acid, which are precursors of the highly active prostaglandins, thromboxanes, leukotrienes, and lipoxins commonly associated with inflammation and thrombosis, as well as with the antithrombotic hormone prostacyclin.

The other fatty acid class is synthesized in small quantities by terrestrial plants and in larger amounts by the aquatic single-cell plants called plankton (Lin et al., 1982). Since plankton is the ultimate food source for all marine fish, the same fatty acids are found in high concentration in their body fat. These acids are characterized by the location of the first of their multiple double bonds three carbon atoms from the methyl end of the side chain, and are therefore called in chemical nomenclature "n-3" or "ω-3" fatty acids. The metabolic oxidation products

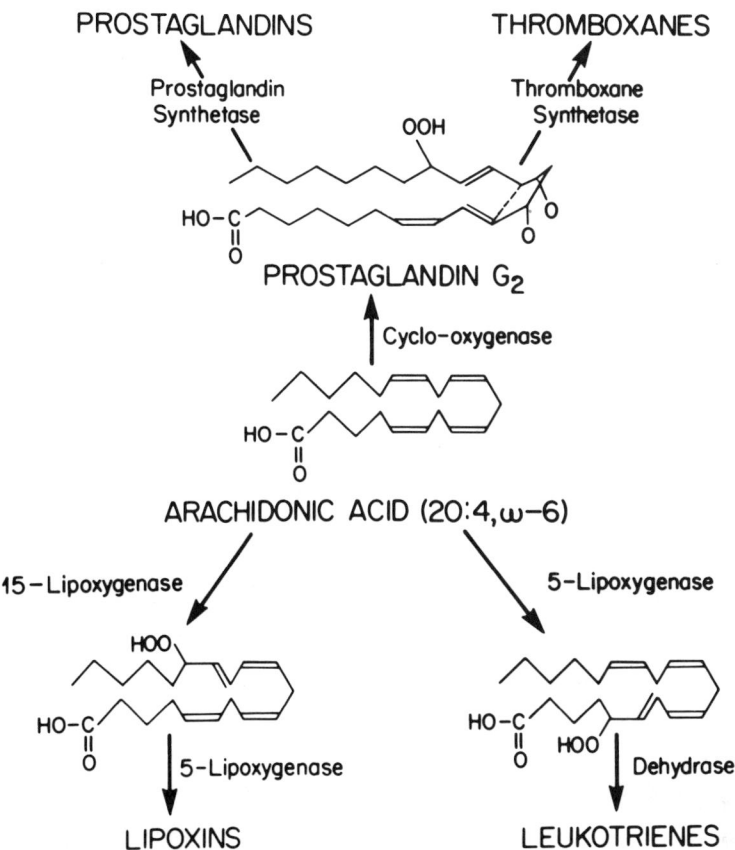

Figure 6 The pathways of oxidative metabolism of arachidonic acid to biologically active products. As discussed in the text, other polyunsaturated fatty acids may be oxidized via the same enzymatic pathways, but the hormone analogs produced have widely varying potency with respect to those produced from arachidonic acid.

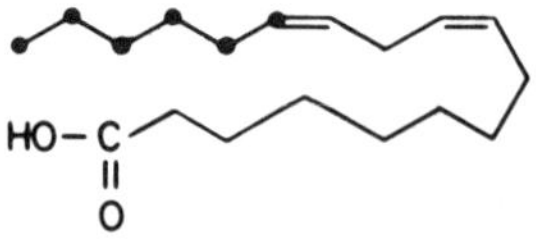

LINOLEIC   ACID   (18:2, ω−6)

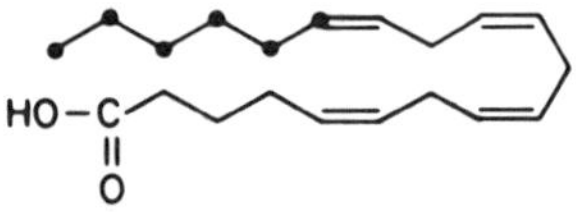

ARACHIDONIC   ACID   (20:4, ω−6)

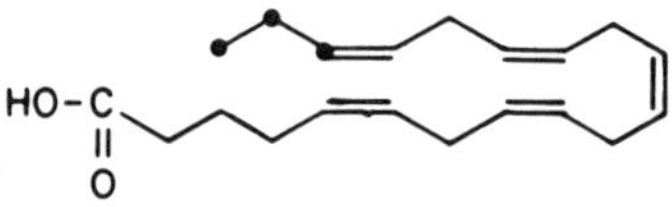

EICOSAPENTAENOIC   ACID = EPA   (20:5, ω−3)

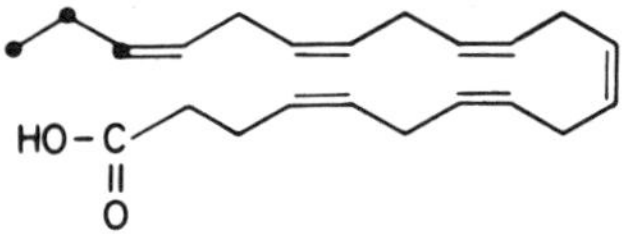

DOCOSAHEXAENOIC   ACID = DHA (22:6, ω−3)

Figure 7 Examples of metabolically important, naturally occurring polyunsaturated fatty acids. The upper two examples have the first double bond six carbon atoms in from the terminal methyl group, while the lower two acids have the first double bond only three carbon atoms in from the methyl end of the molecule. The two classes of fatty acids are not interconvertible in the human body and produce active oxidation products (see Fig. 6) of very different hormonal potency.

of these acids are, in general, much less active than their n-6 counterparts. With respect to cardiovascular disease, for instance, thromboxane A_3, the n-3 analog of the strong blood platelet aggregant and n-6 derivative thromboxane A_2, is almost inactive (Dyerberg et al., 1978). There is an important exception, however, in that PGI_3, the n-3 counterpart of prostacyclin, a strong platelet *disaggregant* synthesized by the vascular endothelium, is almost as potent as the n-6 prostacyclin PGI_2 (Dyerberg et al., 1978, Dyerberg and Bang, 1979). Thus, eating fish fat in quantity, and increasing the human depot fat content of n-3 relative to n-6 fatty acids, should and does (Dyerberg et al., 1978; Dyerberg and Bang, 1979; Glomset, 1985) have a nutritional antithrombotic effect (see Chapter 2).

Similarly, with respect to inflammatory disease, the n-3 fatty acids are less effective substrates for the lipoxygenases (Fig. 6) which convert them into leukotrienes and lipoxins (Lee et al., 1984, Lewis and Austen, 1984) and, in the case of eicosapentaenoic acid (EPA), inhibit the conversion of arachidonic acid into leukotrienes (Lee et al., 1984). These data suggest that fish oil ingestion should modify the inflammatory response, and both animal (Prickett et al., 1981, 1984, Robinson et al., 1986) and recent human (Kremer et al., 1987) studies suggest that such is the case. These data are discussed in much greater detail in Chapter 4.

One last general point concerning dietary fat is that the physical chemistry of dietary fat and, therefore, of depot and membrane fat, is most important to its function. Saturated fats, in general, melt at much higher temperatures than do unsaturated fats. This is true not only of triglycerides, but of cholesterol esters and phospholipids as well. Many highly saturated fats, e.g., cocoa butter, butter, coconut oil, are crystalline or semisolid at room temperature. Since most lipids do not function unless in the liquid state, intake or endogenous synthesis of unsaturated fatty acids is essential for the existence of poikilothermic animals (imagine walking if your own subcutaneous fat had the consistency of a chocolate bar!). At a more subtle level, the physicochemical properties of different fatty acids as major components of cell membranes or plasma lipoproteins may have profound effects on cellular and organismal metabolism. We are only beginning to appreciate some of these effects (Spritz and Mishkel, 1969; Mishkel and Spritz, 1969, Spector and Yorek, 1985; Parks and Bullock, 1987). In the next section, we consider some of the general relationships of dietary fat to human disease, as well as the methods by which these correlations have been elucidated.

DIETARY FAT INTAKE AND DISEASE

This topic is, in a sense, the mirror image of the relationships of dietary fat to human health. We review it here, however, not in physiological terms, as we did in the previous section, but rather in relation to chemical, toxicological, and pathological parameters.

Dietary fat is an important caloric source for human metabolism and the major substrate that keeps us alive during most of each day. In many ways, fat is an almost perfect food. It is widely available, an efficient source of energy at 9 cal/g compared with only 4 for carbohydrate and protein, and can be turned into energy with only minimal metabolic modification. Human beings have existed for centuries on widely varying fat sources, ranging from purely vegetable sources to fat from terrestrial animals to exclusively marine animal fats. This remarkable human adaptability is often forgotten while we concentrate on the problems that sometimes arise from this generally benign food source.

Intrinsic Properties of Dietary Fat in Relation to Disease

Many of the relationships of the intrinsic properties of fat to disease have been alluded to in the previous section. These include the saturation of the dietary fat, its sterol content, total fat intake, and the stereochemistry of the unsaturated fatty acids.

Dietary fat saturation has been the subject of intense study for years, and the interested reader should consult general reviews of the subject (Goodnight et al., 1982; Mattson and Grundy,

1985, McNamara et al., 1987). The purposes of this chapter are best served by a brief summary of current thought. An increase in the saturated fat intake as a percent of total fat intake is associated with an increase in plasma total cholesterol and appears to raise low-density lipoprotine (LDL) and high-density lipoprotein (HDL) cholesterol equally (Grundy, 1986). Epidemiological data link it to an increased incidence of atherosclerotic death (Turpeinen, 1979), and perhaps to certain cancers, although the data on the latter point is, at best, equivocal (Carroll, 1975). However, some of the world's longest-lived populations, on average, eat a high-saturated-fat diet. Furthermore, there may be inverse correlation between plasma cholesterol concentrations and risk of cancer death (e.g., Schatzkin et al., 1987). An increase in the relative proportion of monounsaturated fats in the diet is associated with moderate plasma cholesterol concentrations, with lower LDL, and with relatively high HDL levels (Grundy, 1986). Such a diet, consumed by much of the population of the Mediterranean basin, is associated with a low cardiovascular death rate and has recently been championed (Grundy, 1986) as a healthful alternative to the high-polyunsaturated-fat diet that has been in vogue for some years. The latter diet may or may not lower LDL and HDL cholesterol (Goodnight et al., 1982, Grundy, 1986). It increases biliary cholesterol and has been associated with a higher incidence of both gallstones and cancer in one large epidemiological study (Pearce and Dayton, 1971; Sturdevant et al., 1973). In animal models, polyunsaturated fats may act as tumor promoters (Carroll and Khor, 1975). However, most of these data, human and animal, were obtained with n-6 fatty acids as the dietary source. Of particular note with respect to this discussion is that n-3 fatty acids may behave very differently. In recent studies fish oils have been shown to lower plasma triglycerides and VLDL, with a lesser effect on LDL or HDL concentrations. When fed as the sole fat source, fish produce a pathologically low platelet count and a profound bleeding defect (Dyerberg et al., 1978, Dyerberg and Bang, 1979).

Dietary sterol content seems clearly to be associated with risk of atherosclerotic disease. Not only may a high cholesterol

intake raise plasma cholesterol and be associated with a higher
incidence of atherosclerosis (Quintao et al., 1971, Turpeinen,
1979), but a high plant sterol intake inhibits cholesterol absorption and lowers plasma cholesterol (Lees et al., 1977; Tilvis and
Miettinen, 1986). Diets high in plant sterols are those high in vegetable fat and low in animal fat. Such diets are often high in fiber
and are eaten by populations with low death rates from both atherosclerosis and gastrointestinal cancer. Very recent studies in
Finnish subjects (Kesaniemi et al., 1987) have shown that plasma
apo E phenotype, a readily studied genetic marker, relates directly
to dietary cholesterol absorption, endogenous cholesterol synthesis, and plasma cholesterol concentration. Genetically determined responsiveness to dietary cholesterol intake is almost certainly generally true in humans since the relationship of apo E
phenotype to plasma cholesterol concentration is a worldwide
phenomenon (Utermann et al., 1984; Sing and Davignon, 1985).

      As noted above, the relationship between marine sterol in-
take and disease is complex. Fish and crustacea contain cholesterol, and some fish oils contain a lot of cholesterol, while mollusks contain both cholesterol and a number of other sterols
that may behave like cholesterol. The net effect of mollusk
sterols on plasma cholesterol appears to be negligible. Diets
very high in plant or marine sterols run the risk of raising their
levels in plasma (Lees and Lees, 1976) even in normal subjects,
and in certain patients may produce serious illness (Bhattacharyya and Connor, 1974, Salen et al., 1985b, Gregg et al., 1986).

      The relationship of total fat intake to disease is complex;
in most studies on fat intake, saturated or unsaturated fat or
sterol intake, rather than total fat, has been correlated with a
particular disease. It is not clear that a high total fat intake, per
se, is particularly related to any disease.

      Finally, and most important to the theme of this book, the
fine structure of the unsaturated fatty acids in the diet is important. The prescient studies of Spritz and Mishkel in the 1960s
(Spritz and Mishkel, 1969; Mishkel and Spritz, 1969) are illustra-
tive of this point. Spritz hypothesized that many of the effects of
unsaturated fatty acids were related to their cross-sectional area

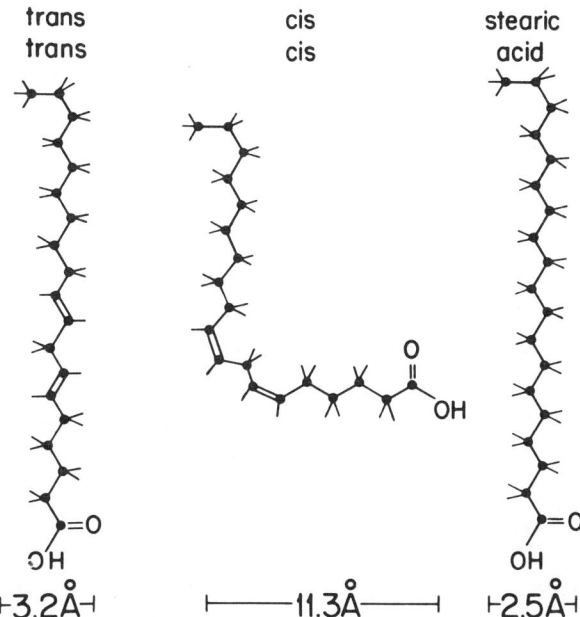

Figure 8 The cross-sectional area of two stereoisomeric linoleic acids. The fully saturated analog stearic acid is included for comparison. The lateral cross-sectional area of the normally occurring *cis-cis* linoleic acid is much greater than that of the *trans-trans* linoleic acid produced by in vitro hydrogenation. The latter is not only structurally similar to stearic acid (see text), but behaves metabolically in an anomalous way. See text for details.

(Fig. 8). Because the normal *cis* double bond bends the fatty acid chain at roughly a 120° angle, the presence of one double bond increases the area occupied by that chain; multiple double bonds increase its cross-sectional area even more. Spritz postulated that the cholesterol-lowering effects of polyunsaturated fatty acids were related to their "bulk" and that the percent lipid lowering should be directly related to the ratio of the cross-sectional area of the polyunsaturated fatty acids to that of the saturated dietary fatty acids fed as a control. The investigators then performed human feeding studies to prove their point and showed

that the expected change did occur both for LDL and for HDL
(Spritz and Mishkel, 1969). This was perhaps the first study to
show that polyunsaturated fat feeding lowered HDL cholesterol
as well as LDL cholesterol.

Spritz and his colleagues went much further, however. They
realized that all-*trans* polyunsaturated fatty acids have virtually
the same cross-sectional area as saturated fatty acids (Fig. 8) and
postulated that triglycerides made from such acids should not
lower plasma lipids, *despite their great unsaturation*. Then they
put their hypothesis to the test. They had custom-synthesized for
them a relatively large amount of *trans trans* trilinolein and fed
it as the sole fat source to a series of human volunteers.

The results considerably exceeded their expectations. Not
only did the subjects' plasma lipids not decrease, they increased
dramatically, and after a few weeks of the *trans* fatty acid diet the
subjects themselves developed a severe and painful peripheral
neuropathy, which slowly subsided when they resumed a normal
diet (Mishkel and Spritz, 1969). Needless to say, the human studies were stopped at that point, and definitive data on the cause of
the neuropathy were never obtained. Subsequent studies with
mono-*trans* fatty acids, which are present in moderate amounts in
partially hydrogenated vegetable oils, did not reproduce the toxic
effects seen with the *trans trans* acid (Mattson et al., 1975).
Nevertheless, Spritz's studies dramatically highlighted the importance of the structure and isomerism of dietary fatty acids and set
the stage for the more recent findings on the metabolic differences
between the n-6 and n-3 isomers.

Extrinsic Considerations

Disease may be caused by many factors extrinsic to the major
and minor constituents that are expected to be in the dietary fat.
These extrinsic agents include naturally derived toxins such as
mycotoxins—compounds that contaminate dietary fat secondary
to fungal growth on the fat or on the food from which the fat is
extracted. Aflatoxin, a highly potent carcinogen synthesized by
the fungus *Aspergillus flavus*, is an almost constant, but usually

low-level contaminant of peanuts and therefore of peanut oil
(Wogan and Busby, 1980). Keeping the level of this fat-soluble
toxin within prescribed limits requires constant monitoring of the
supplies of this widely used food fat. Other kinds of food spoilage
may introduce toxic ingredients—oxidation of polyunsaturated fat
may introduce lipid peroxides which may be atherogenic and
mutagenic (Carroll, 1975). Environmental toxins readily enter
the food chain. Hydrocarbons such as benzpyrene, insecticides
like DDT, industrial agents such as PCBs, to name some well-
known toxins, may be found in increasing concentrations in marine animals as one ascends the food chain from marine plants to
predatory fish like bluefish and striped bass (McEwen and Stephenson, 1979).

A third class of extrinsic food contaminants that may cause
disease is food additivies, in this case agents added to food to prevent spoilage or rancidity of fat. The most widely used additives
or preservatives in the past were butylated hydroxytoluene (BHT)
and butylated hydroxyanisole (BHA), both phenolic antioxidants
(Coppen, 1983). However, both BHA and BHT may be tumor
promoters, and perhaps even carcinogens (Shamberger, 1983),
and their allowable concentration in foods is limited. Interestingly, in other studies, BHA and BHT have been shown to inhibit
mutagenesis, probably because of their antioxidant properties.
Similarly, tocopherols, i.e., vitamin E, which are natural antioxidant phenols in food fat, inhibit mutagenesis, are sometimes used
as food additives, and are perhaps the safest in terms of preventing
rather than causing disease (Loliger, 1983).

In summary, although it seems clear that a high-cholesterol,
high-saturated-fat diet raises plasma lipids and probably thereby
increases the risk of atherosclerosis, there is little evidence that the
kind of food fat eaten produces other human disease, except
through spoilage, environmental toxins, either natural or man-
made, and perhaps food additives. The tremendous adaptability
of the human organism to its dietary caloric sources allows us
to remain healthy over a wide range of diet. Whether certain
chronic diseases such as arteriosclerosis, cancer, or arthritis can be
prevented or ameliorated, which is a somewhat different question,
is the topic of the remainder of this chapter and this volume.

Clues to Disease Etiology in Relation to Dietary Fat

A number of hypotheses have been generated, and some notable
conclusions reached, from studies designed either to generate or
to test certain clues to the relationship between fat intake and human disease. These almost all fall into two categories—experimental pathology, i.e., studies with animal models of human disease,
and epidemiology, i.e., studies of large numbers of people to determine certain associations of dietary habits and disease. Some of
the latter studies have been based on observation alone, with a
careful attempt made *not* to affect the population studied, or they
were retrospective, in which case different problems arose. Other
epidemiological studies have been interventional, in which a large
number of individuals are fed one diet and a matched group
another, and the occurrence of disease in the two groups compared. In some of these studies, the two groups are switched in
the middle of the study, so that each can serve as its own control.

It is well beyond the scope of this introductory chapter even
to review in brief the enormous number of animal studies on fat
and disease and the almost as large number of human studies. We
will note some general advantages and disadvantages of these types
of study, cite a few pertinent examples, and leave the details for
subsequent chapters.

Experimental pathology has many attractive features. An
animal model whose metabolism is similar to that of humans can
be chosen, and conditions fixed as far as possible with only a
single variable. The animals can be sacrificed and a complete
pathological evaluation performed. Perhaps the major problem
is that all the diseases under discussion are chronic diseases often
evident late in life, 30 or more years after the beginning of exposure to the diet in question. Since the animals most similar to
humans are also long-lived, the cost of appropriate studies becomes prohibitive. In most cases, either the intervention is esca-
lated to an unphysiological level so that the desired end point is
reached in a much shorter time, or a shorter-lived animal species
is used, so that chronic disease appears in a convenient time frame.
In either case, the extrapolation of the results to the naturally occurring disease becomes uncertain and may often be quite mislead-

ing. An interesting example is a recent study on the effects of cod liver oil feeding in cholesterol- and saturated-fat-fed swine (Weiner, et al., 1986). Coronary atherosclerosis, which ordinarily occurs in old age in the pig, was accelerated not only by feeding a 2.4% cholesterol-lard-based diet, but also by balloon abrasion of the left anterior descending coronary artery after 3 weeks of the test diet. The animals were killed at 8 months, and all three coronary arteries examined. There was much less atherosclerotic coronary artery disease in four pigs fed 30 ml cod liver oil daily plus the diet than in seven animals fed the atherogenic diet alone. On the face of it, it would seem that cod liver oil feeding is anti-atherogenic. However, that conclusion is probably not supported by the evidence. Not only are the numbers of animals small and the diet most unphysiological for either pigs or humans, but the control diet resulted in undetectable levels of n-3 fatty acids in the animals' blood plasma, and its very high cholesterol content minimized the effects of the large amount of cholesterol ingested in the cod liver oil. Thus, as attractive as this experimental study is, it does not necessarily follow that human subjects on mixed diet would benefit from fish oil supplements, *nor do the authors suggest it*. Unfortunately, these fine points have not always been brought out in the descriptions of this work in the popular press.

Epidemiological studies similarly have many attractive features. When performed prospectively, observational studies have minimal bias, and intervention studies may allow the investigators to determine the effects of a single parameter on the incidence of disease. It is feasible to design studies of long duration; 5 years or even 10 is not rare. No extrapolation from animals to humans is needed.

In many ways, the promise of epidemiological studies has been fulfilled. Much of what we consider to be true about dietary fat and human disease is based on prospective, and occasionally retrospective, human studies. The extensive follow-up of the dramatic increase in coronary disease deaths in Jews migrating from the Arab world to Israel, which coincided, among many other changes, with an increase in their caloric intake (Cohen et al., 1961), the experience of the Finnish and Norwegian popula-

tions during World War II, where a tremendous drop in caloric
intake was paralleled by a similar drop in cardiovascular deaths
(Turpeinen, 1979), the Framingham study (Anderson et al.,
1987), and the interpopulation diet-heart disease data nicely summarized by Turpeinen (Turpeinen, 1979)—all helped to convince
us that dietary fat as well as total calories are directly related to
the causes and progression of human atherosclerosis. Although
the data is much less clear-cut, the prospective dietary intervention
study of the late Seymour Dayton and his colleagues (Dayton
et al., 1969; Pearce and Dayton, 1971; Sturdevant et al., 1973), as
well as recent (Schatzkin et al., 1987) and earlier studies (Armstrong and Doll, 1975; Garcia-Palmieri et al., 1981; Kagan et al.,
1981), suggest that there might be a relationship among dietary
fat intake, serum cholesterol, and some, but not all, cancers in
human populations.

However, the epidemiological approach, too, has many and
serious problems. Retrospective studies may have serious built-
in biases which often invalidate their results. An obvious one is
that those who have died cannot be tested and that the survivors
themselves may be different in important parameters than they
were at an earlier, perhaps critical, time. Prospective observational
studies may suffer from insufficient spontaneous range of variation in the parameter to be studied. For instance, the lack of correlation between dietary cholesterol intake and cardiovascular
death in the Framingham study has been attributed to the narrow
range of cholesterol intakes in that population, which may not
have been wide enough to be meaningful (Connor and Connor,
1972). Intervention studies are particularly susceptible to ambi-
valence. A negative result may mean only that the intended intervention did not accomplish its goal. A positive result may be from
an *unintended* change which accompanied the *intended* intervention. Diet studies that involve exchange of saturated fat for unsaturated fat also exchange animal sterols for plant sterols, as well
as the trace constitutents of each fat source. Any observed effects
of diet could result not from the fat saturation, but rather from
one or more of the other ingredients in the fat. Despite all these
problems, however, the epidemiological approach has remained

one of the most useful methods for determining the effects of
dietary fat on health.

In the last section of this chapter, we briefly examine the
three major diseases to which dietary fat has been linked and attempt to integrate what we have learned from the biochemical,
physiological, pathological and epidemiological considerations reviewed above.

DIETARY FAT AND INDIVIDUAL DISEASES

Cardiovascular Disease

The major cardiovascular disease is atherosclerosis, which is responsible for more deaths by far in the developed countries than
any other disease. As abundantly documented above, dietary fat
quality, as well as quantity, has been linked to the total plasma
cholesterol and the LDL and HDL cholesterol, major risk factors
for atherosclerosis, as well as directly with the incidence of atherosclerotic complications (Leren, 1966, Lipid Research Clinics Program, 1984). Increased intake of saturated fat and cholesterol
is clearly associated with higher plasma lipids and higher risk of
atherosclerosis, while intake of vegetable fat as the major fat
source appears to be associated with lower lipids and less atherosclerosis. These epidemiological conclusions are supported by a
considerable body of biochemical and physiological evidence concerning the effects of fat saturation and particularly cholesterol
intake on plasma cholesterol concentration.

The last decade has seen the rapid accumulation of information concerning the special effects of marine fat on plasma lipids and atherosclerosis. Epidemiologically, high fish consumption
has been associated with low death rates from coronary artery
disease (Dyerberg et al., 1978, Dyerberg and Bang, 1979), although a recent study has suggested that eating fish as little as
twice a week is associated with a meaningful decrease in coronary
disease death (Kromhout et al., 1985). These studies are fraught
with the dangers alluded to above and have stimulated considerable discussion concerning their shortcomings (Bang and Dyerberg, 1985, Curb and Reed, 1985, Greaves et al., 1985; Meydani
et al., 1985; Shekelle et al., 1985; Vollset et al., 1985). Biochem-

ical and physiological findings concerning marine fatty acids are perhaps more convincing, but the effects are seen only when n-3 fatty acids are a significant fraction of total fat intake (Phillipson et al., 1985; Weiner et al., 1986; Parks and Bullock, 1987). These effects include lowering of plasma triglycerides with little effect on LDL and HDL, inhibition of platelet function with prolongation of the bleeding time, and inhibition of granulocyte and monocyte function (Glomset, 1985). Given that monocyte-macrophages are thought to participate actively in atherogenesis (Faggiotto et al., 1984), inhibition of monocyte function may be an important new mechanism of action of antiatherosclerotic agents (Glomset, 1985). These data are reviewed in detail in Chapters 2, 4, and 6.

Cancer

The data on dietary fat and cancer are both less conclusive and less systematized than those concerning atherosclerosis. Epidemiologically, the incidence of breast cancer has been related to the intake of animal fat and total fat (Carroll, 1975; Phillips, 1975), and that of gastrointestinal cancer to total fat intake (Carroll and Khor, 1975; Wynder and Reddy, 1977) and intake of unsaturated fat (Dayton, 1969; Pearce and Dayton, 1971), but also to serum cholesterol and beta-lipoprotein levels (Tömberg et al., 1986). However, in prospective studies (Phillips, 1983; Willett et al., 1987), these findings have not been confirmed. Biochemically, unsaturated fats, at least n-6 fatty acids, may be tumor promoters (Carroll, 1975), and bile acids may be as well (Wynder and Reddy, 1977; Hill et al., 1987). Furthermore, several of the common environmental contaminants, such as PCBs, are carcinogenic. The significance of these findings is discussed in Chapter 5.

Arthritis

There is relatively little epidemiological evidence, to this writer's knowledge, concerning dietary fat intake and arthritic diseases. In contrast, there is a large amount of recent biochemical data which suggests that increasing dietary n-3 fatty acids has an effect on the mechanisms of inflammation, which involve prostaglandins, on the mechanisms of inflammation, which involve prostaglandins, leukotrienes, and lipoxins (Lewis and Austen, 1984, Samuelsson et al., 1987). In one experimental animal study this effect was to exacerbate arthritis (Prickett et al., 1984). In a recent clinical study of 33 patients with rheumatoid arthritis, daily administration of 15 g of fish oil as a diet supplement was associated within 3 months with subjective and objective improvement in multiple parameters, including joint tenderness and swelling. Since the study was conducted on a double-blind basis, the results warrant careful consideration. The data on dietary fat intake and arthritis are reviewed in detail in Chapter 4.

CONCLUSION

Although human beings are remarkably adaptable in their ability to remain healthy over a wide range of dietary fat sources and intakes, the fat in the diet is clearly associated with the occurrence of, or freedom from, certain diseases. The evidence is particularly strong for coronary heart disease, and less so for cancer. Although little is known about the effects of dietary fat on arthritic and rheumatic diseases, the available evidence suggests that the nature of the dietary fat may be therapeutically important in these syndromes. In all these areas, the recent emergence of dietary polyunsaturated fat as a precursor of potent metabolic intermediates has radically changed our concepts of the potential mechanisms of diet-induced effects on health and disease. In particular, the therapeutic effects of dietary fat changes in disease may be significant, even though health may be maintained over a wide range of intakes. In this regard, the recent findings that certain fish oil fatty acids, the n-3 polyunsaturated acids, are synthesized into eicosanoids with significantly different metabolic effects than those from the n-6 fatty acids lends a powerful rationale to this concept. Subsequent chapters review the details of the effects of marine fat on health and the mechanics and problems of supplying these products to the food and pharmaceutical industries.

REFERENCES

Anderson KM, Castelli WP, Levy D. Cholesterol and mortality. 30 years of follow-up from the Framingham study. JAMA 1987;257:2176-2180.

Armstrong B, Doll R. Environmental factors and cancer incidence and mortality in different countries, with special reference to dietary practices. Int J Cancer 1975;15:617-631.

Assmann G. Lipid Metabolism and atherosclerosis. Stuttgart, New York. Schattauer, 1982.

Bang HO, Dyerberg J. Fish consumption and mortality from coronary heart disease (Letter to the Editor). N Engl J Med 1985;313:822-823.

Bhattacharyya AK, Connor WE. Beta-sitosterolemia and xanthomatosis: a newly described lipid storage disease in two sisters. J Clin Invest 1974;53:1033-1043.

Borgstrom B. Quantification of cholesterol absorption in man by fecal analysis after the feeding of a single isotope-labeled meal. J Lipid Res 1979;10:331-337.

Borgstrom B, Erlanson-Albertsson C, Wieloch T. Pancreatic colipase: chemistry and physiology. J Lipid Res 1979;20:805-816.

Cahill GF Jr, Herrera MG, Morgan AP, et al. Hormone-fuel interrelationships during fasting. J Clin Invest 1966;45:1751-1769.

Carey MC. The enterohepatic circulation. In: Arias I, Schachter D, Shafritz DA, eds. The liver: biology and pathobiology. New York, Raven Press, 1982; 429-465.

Carroll KK. Experimental evidence of dietary factors and hormone-dependent cancers. Cancer Res 1975;35:3374-3383.

Carroll KK, Khor HT. Experimental evidence of dietary factors and hormone-dependent cancers. Cancer Res 1975;35:3374-3383.

Cohen AM, Bavly S, Poznanski R. Change of diet of Yemenite Jews in relation to diabetes and ischaemic heart-disease. Lancet 1961;2:1399-1401.

Connor, WE, Connor SL. The key role of nutritional factors in the prevention of coronary heart disease. Prev Med 1972; 1:49-83.

Connor WE, Lin SE. Absorption and transport of shellfish sterols in human subjects. Gastroenterology 1981;81:276-284.

Connor WE, Lin SE. The effect of shellfish in the diet upon the plasma lipid levels in humans. Metab Clin Exp 1982;31: 1046-1051.

Coppen PP. The use of antioxidants. In Allen JC, Hamilton RJ, eds. Rancidity in foods. London: Applied Science Publishers 1983; 67-87.

Crouse JR, Grundy SM, Ahrens EH Jr. Cholesterol distribution in the bulk tissues of man: variation with age. J Clin Invest 1972;51:1292-1296.

Curb JD, Reed DM. Fish consumption and mortality from coronary heart disease (Letter to the Editor). N Engl J Med 1985;313:821.

Dayton S, Pearce MI, Hashimoto S, et al. A controlled clinical trial of a diet high in unsaturated fat in preventing complications of atherosclerosis. Circulation 1969;40(Suppl II).

Dyerberg J, Bang HO. Haemostatic function and platelet polyunsaturated fatty acids in eskimos. Lancet 1979;2:433-435.

Dyerberg J, Bang HO, Stoffersen E, et al. Eicosapentaenoic acid and prevention of thrombosis and atherosclerosis? Lancet 1978;2:117-119.

Faggiotto A, Ross R, Harker L. Studies of hypercholesterolemia in the nonhuman primate I. Changes that lead to fatty-streak formation. Arteriosclerosis 1984;4:323-340.

Fredrickson DS, Gordon RS. Transport of fatty acids. Physiol Rev 1958;38:585-630.

Fritz IB. Factors influencing the rates of long chain fatty acid oxidation and synthesis in mammalian systems. Physiol Rev 1961;41:52-129.

Gage SH. The free granules (chylomicrons) of the blood as shown by the dark-field microscope. Cornell Veterinarian 1920; 10:154-155.

Gage SH and Fish PA. Fat digestion and assimilation in man and animals as determined by dark field microscope and fat-soluble dye. Amer J Anatomy 1924;34:1-85.

Garcia-Palmieri MR, Sorlie PD, Costas R, et al. An apparent inverse relationship between serum cholesterol and cancer mortality in Puerto Rico. Am J Epidemiol 1981;114:29-40.

Glomset JA. Fish, fatty acids, and human health (Editorial). N Engl J Med 1985;312:1253-1254.

Goodman DS. The interaction of human serum albumin with long-chain fatty acid anions. J Am Chem Soc 1958;80:3892-3898.

Goodnight SH, Harris WS, Connor WE, Illingworth DR. Polyunsaturated fatty acids, hyperlipidemia and thrombosis. Arteriosclerosis 1982;2:87-113.

Gould RG, Jones RJ, LeRoy GV, Wissler RW, Taylor CB. Absorbability of beta-sitosterol in humans. Metabolism 1969;18:652-662.

Greaves M, Cartwright IJ, Pickley AG, et al. Fish consumption and mortality from coronary heart disease (Letter to the Editor). N Engl J Med 1985;313:822.

Gregg, RE, Connor WE, Lin DS, Brewer HB. Abnormal metabolism of shellfish sterols in a patient with sitosterolemia and xanthomatosis. J Clin Invest 1986;77:1864-1872.

Grundy SM. Comparison of monounsaturated fatty acids and carbohydrates for lowering plasma cholesterol. N Engl J Med 1986;324:745-748.

Havel RJ, Goldstein JL, Brown MS. Lipoproteins and lipid transport. In Bondy PK, Rosenberg LE, eds. Metabolic control and disease. Philadelphia: Saunders, 1980; 393-494.

Hill MJ, Melville DM, Lennard-Jones JE, Neale K, Ritchie JK. Faecal bile acids, dysplasia and carcinoma in ulcerative colitis. Lancet 1987;2:185-186.

Hofmann AF. Chemistry and enterohepatic circulation of bile acids. Hepatology 1984;4(Suppl):45-145.

Hofmann AF, Molino G, Milanese M, Belforte G. Description and simulation of a physiological pharmacokinetic model for the metabolism and enterohepatic circulation of bile acids in man. J Clin Invest 1983;71:1003-1022.

Kagan A, McGee DL, Yano K, et al. Serum cholesterol and mortality in a Japanese-American population: the Honolulu Heart Program. Am J Epidemiol 1981,114:29-40.

Kesaniemi YA, Ehnholm C, Miettinen TA. Intestinal cholesterol absorption efficiency in man is related to apoprotein E phenotype. J Clin Invest 1987;80:578-581.

Kermer JM, Jubiz W, Michalek A, et al. Fish-oil fatty acid supplementation in active rheumatoid arthritis. Ann Intern Med 1987;106:497-503.

Kromhout D, Bosschieter EB, Coulander C. The inverse relation between fish consumption and 20-year mortality from coronary heart disease. N Engl J Med 1985;312:1205-1209.

Lee TH, Mencia-Huerta JM, Shih C, et al. Effects of exogenous arachidonic, eicosapentaenoic, and docosahexaenoic acids on the generation of 5-lipoxygenase pathway products by ionophore-activated human neutrophils. J Clin Invest 1984;74:1922-1924.

Lees AM, Mok HYI, Lees RS, et al. Plant sterols as cholesterol-lowering agents: clinical trials in patients with hypercholestrolemia and studies of sterol balance. Atherosclerosis 1977;28:325-338.

Lees RS, Lees AM. Effects of sitosterol therapy on plasma lipid and lipoprotein composition. In Greten H, ed. Lipoprotein metabolism. Berlin: Springer-Verlag 1976, 119-124.

Leren P. The effect of plasma cholesterol lowering diet in male survivors of myocaridal infarction. A controlled clinical trial. Oslo Universitetsforlaget, 1966.

Lewis B. The hyperlipidaemias. London: Blackwell Scientific Publications 1976.

Lewis RA, Austen KF. The biologically active leukotrienes. Biosynthesis, metabolism, receptors, functions and pharmacology. J Clin Invest 1984;73:889-897.

Lin DS, Ilias AM, Connor WE, et al. Composition and biosynthesis of sterols in selected marine phytoplankton. Lipids 1982; 17:818-824.

Lin DS, Connor WE, Phillipson BE. Sterol composition of normal human bile, effect of feeding shellfish (marine) sterols. Gastroenterology 1984;86:611-617.

Lipid Research Clinics Program. The Lipid Research Clinics Coronorary Primary Prevention Trial results: I. Reduction in incidence of coronary heart disease. JAMA 1984;251:351-364.

Loliger J. Natural oxidants. In Allen JC, Hamilton RJ, eds. Rancidity in foods. London: Applied Science Publishers, 1983; 89-107.

Machlin LJ, ed. Handbook of vitamins. Nutritional, biochemical and clinical aspects. New York: Dekker, 1984.

Mattson FH, Grundy SM. Comparison of effects of dietary saturated, monounsaturated, and polyunsaturated fatty acids on plasma lipids and lipoproteins in man. J Lipid Res 1985; 26:194-202.

Mattson FH, Hollenbach EJ, Kligman AM. Effect of hydrogenated fat on the plasma cholesterol and triglyceride levels of man. Am J Clin Nutr 1975;28:726-731.

McEwen FL, Stephenson GR. The use and significance of pesticides in the environment, Chapter 15. New York: Wiley, 1979; 260-348.

McGiff JC. Thromboxane and prostacyclin: implications for function and disease of the vasculature. Adv Intern Med 1980;25:199-216.

McNamara DJ, Kolb R, Parker TS, et al. Heterogeneiety of cholesterol homeostasis in man. Response to changes in dietary fat quality and cholesterol quantity. J Clin Invest 1987; 79:1729-1739.

Meydani SN, Siguel E, Shapiro AC, Blumberg JB. Fish consumption and mortality from coronary heart disease (Letter to the Editor). N Engl J Med 1985;313:822.

Mishkel MA, Spritz N. The effects of trans isomerized trilinolein on plasma lipids of man. In: Holmes WL, Carlson LA, Paoletti R, eds. Advances in experimental medicine and biology. New York: Plenum Press, 1969; 355-364.

Nestel PJ, Connor WE, Reardon MF, et al. Suppression by diets rich in fish oil of very low density lipoprotine production in man. J Clin Invest 1984;74:82-89.

Parks JS, Bullock BC. Effect of fish oil versus lard diets on the chemical and physical properties of low density lipoproteins of nonhuman primates. J Lipid Res 1987;28:173-182.

Pearce ML, Dayton S. Incidence of cancer in men on a diet high in polyunsaturated fat. Lancet 1971;1:464-467.

Phillips RL. Role of life-style and dietary habits in risk of cancer among Seventh-Day Adventists. Cancer Res 1975;35:3513-3522.

Phillips RL, Snowdon DA. Association of meat and coffee use with cancers of the large bowel, breast, and prostate among Seventh-Day Adventists: Preliminary results. Cancer Res 1983;43(5 suppl):2403s-2408s.

Phillipson BE, Rothrock DW, Connor WE, et al. Reduction of plasma lipids, lipoproteins, and apoproteins by dietary fish oils in patients with hypertriglyceridemia. N Engl J Med 1985;312:1210-1216.

Poland A, Knutson JC. 2,3,7,8 Tetrachlorodibenzo-p-dioxin and related halogenated aromatic hydrocarbons: examination of the mechanism of toxicity. Annu Rev Pharmacol Toxicol 1982;22:517-554.

Prickett JD, Robinson DR, Steinberg AD. Dietary enrichment with the polyunsaturated fatty acid eicosapentaenoic acid prevents proteinuria and prolongs survival in (NZB $\times$ NZW) F_1 mice. J Clin Invest 1981;68:556-559.

Prickett JD, Trentham DE, Robinson DR. Dietary fish oil augments the induction of arthritis in rats immunized with type II collagen. J Immunol 1984;132:725-729.

Quintao E, Grundy SM, Ahrens EH Jr. Effects of dietary cholesterol on the regulation of total body cholesterol in man.
J Lipid Res 1971;12:233.

Reis GJ, Boucher TM, Sipperly ME, Silverman DI, McCabe CH,
Bain DS, Sacks FM, Grossman W, Pasternak RC. Randomized trial of fish oil for prevention of restenosis after coronary angioplasty. Lancet 1989;2:177-181.

Robinson DR, Prickett JD, Makoul GT, Steinberg AD, Colvin RB.
Dietary fish oil reduces progression of established renal
disease in (NZB X NZW) F_1 mice and delays renal disease
in BXSB and MRL/1 strains. Arthritis Rheum 1986;29:539-
546.

Salen G, Ahrens EH Jr, Grundy SM. Metabolism of beta-sitosterol
in man. J Clin Invest 1970;49:952-967.

Salen G, Hora I, Rothkopf M, et al. Lethal atherosclerosis associated with abnormal plasma and tissue sterol composition in
sitosterolemia with xanthomatosis. J Lipid Res 1985a;26:
1126-1133.

Salen G, Kwiterovich S, Shefer S, et al. Increased plasma choles-
tanol and 5α-saturated plant sterol derivatives in subjects with
sitosterolemia and xanthomatosis. J Lipid Res 1985b;26:
203-209.

Samuelsson B, Dahlen S-E, Lindgren J, Rouzer CA, Serhan CN.
Leukotrienes and lipoxins: structures, biosynthesis, and biological effects. Science 1987;237:1171-1176.

Schatzkin A, Taylor PR, Carter CL, et al. Serum cholesterol and
cancer in the NHANES I epidemiologic followup study.
Lancet 1987;2:298-301.

Semeriva M, Desnuelle P. Pancreatic lipase and colipase. An example of heterogeneous biocatalysis. Adv Enzymol 1979;
48:319-370.

Shamberger RJ. Nutrition and cancer. New York, London:
Plenum Press, 1983; 313-316.

Shekelle RB, Missell LV, Paul O, et al. Fish consumption and
mortality from coronary heart disease (Letter to the Editor). N Engl J Med 1985;313:820.

Sing CF, Davignon J. Role of the apolipoprotein E polymorphism in determining normal plasma lipid and lipoprotein variation. Am J Hum Genet 1985;37:268-285.

Spector AA. Fatty acid binding to plasma albumin. J Lipid Res 1975;16:165-179.

Spector AA, Yorek MA. Membrane lipid composition cellular function. J Lipid Res 1985;26:1015-1035.

Spritz N, Mishkel MA. Effects of dietary fats on plasma lipids and lipoproteins: an hypothesis for the lipid-lowering effect of unsaturated fatty acids. J Clin Invest 1969;48:78-86.

Stenson WF, Parker CW. Leukotrienes. Adv Intern Med 1984; 30:175-199.

Sturdevant RAJ, Pearce ML, Dayton S. Increased prevalence of cholelithiasis in men ingesting a serum-cholesterol lowering diet. N Engl J Med 1973;288:24-27.

Tilvis RS, Miettinen TA. Serum plant sterols and their relation to cholesterol absorption. Am J Clin Nutr 1986;43:92-97.

Törnberg SA, Holm LE, Carstenson JM, Eklund GA. Risks of cancer of the colon and rectum in relation to serum cholesterol and beta-lipoprotein. N Engl J Med 1986;315:1629-1638.

Turpeinen O. Effect of cholesterol-lowering diet on mortality from coronary heart disease and other causes. Circulation 1979;59:1-7.

Utermann GI, Kindermann I, Kaffarnik H, Steinmetz A. Apolipoprotein E phenotypes and hyperlipidemia. Hum Genet 1984;65:232-236.

Vollset SE, Heuch I, Bjelke E. Fish consumption and mortality from coronary heart disease (Letter to the Editor). N Engl J Med 1985;313:820-821.

Weiner BH, Ockene IS, Levine PH, et al. Inhibition of atherosclerosis by cod-liver oil in a hyperlipidemic swine model. N Engl J Med 1986;315:842-846.

Willett WC, Stampfer MJ, Colditz GA, et al. Dietary fat and the risk of breast cancer. N Engl J Med 1987;316:22-28.

Wogan GN, Busby WF Jr. Naturally occurring carcinogens. In Liener IE, ed. Toxic constituents of plant foodstuffs. New York: Academic Press, 1980; 329-369.

Wynder EL, Reddy BS. Diet and cancer of the colon. In Winick M, ed. Nutrition and cancer. New York: Wiley, 1977; 55-71.

2
Effects of Omega-3 Fatty Acids on Risk Factors for Cardiovascular Disease

D. Roger Illingworth and Daniel Ullmann
Oregon Health Sciences University
Portland, Oregon

INTRODUCTION

Epidemiological studies in several populations, including Greenland Eskimos and fishermen in Japan, have indicated that habitual consumption of a diet enriched in fish or products from other marine animals is associated with a lower incidence of cardiovascular disease than occurs in similar populations in whom the daily intake of marine products is low (Bang et al., 1976; Kagawa et al., 1982, Kromhout et al., 1985). These epidemiological data have been interpreted to indicate that diets containing fish and other marine animals, such as seals, may favorably influence known risk factors for the development of atherosclerosis. Many factors are known to influence the progression of atherosclerosis; these include hypertension, cigarette smoking, diabetes mellitus, hypercholesterolemia, and a positive family history for coronary heart disease. In addition, factors promoting platelet aggregation or endothelial injury and elevated levels of fibrinogen may also accelerate the development of the atherosclerotic process (Ross, 1986, Steinberg, 1987). The present chapter reviews data on the influence of diets containing increased amounts of omega-3 fatty acids, either as constituents of fish or as fish oils, on the plasma concentrations of cholesterol, triglyceride, and individual lipoproteins, platelet function and parameters of hemostasis, blood pressure, and control of diabetes. We focus on studies involving human subjects, but as a background, we briefly review data from animal studies in which the influence of fish oils on the development of experimental atherosclerosis has been examined.

DIETARY OMEGA-3 FATTY ACIDS AND ATHEROSCLEROSIS

The usefulness of animals, particularly rabbits, dogs, and monkeys, for the study of experimental atherosclerosis has been well demonstrated over the last several decades. Diet-induced hyperlipidemia has been associated with the progressive development of arteriosclerosis, which can be reversed upon lowering the plasma lipid concentrations by feeding animals a diet low in cholesterol and generally low in saturated fat. The influence of dietary supplementation with fish oils on experimental atherosclerosis has been the subject of several recent studies. Casali et al. (1986) compared graft patency in three groups of dogs, one a control group fed regular dog chow, a second group fed mackerel supplemented with menhaden oil, and the third group receiving regular dog chow but also receiving dipyridamole and aspirin. Bleeding times were significantly prolonged in the fish oil and aspirin plus dipyridamole-treated dogs as compared with control animals, although in vitro indices of platelet aggregation did not differ. Concentrations of total cholesterol and individual lipoproteins were also similar in all three groups, but when the animals were sacrificed after 6 months on the diet, 86% of the grafts in the fish oil-fed animals remained patent as compared to only 44% in the control group. The patency rate was 79% in the dipyridamole plus aspirin-treated dogs. The authors also noted a significant reduction of intimal thickening in the dogs on the fish oil-containing diet as compared with animals in the control group or the dogs fed the control diet plus dipyridamole and aspirin. The authors concluded that the improved graft patency in the dogs on the fish oil-containing diet was attributable to favorable effects of the omega-3 fatty acids on platelet function and on the proliferation of the atherosclerotic plaque. Plasma concentrations of total cholesterol remained below 160 mg/dl in all three groups of animals, and the development of hyperlipidemia does not appear to be a confounding variable in this study.

In a recent study, Weiner et al. (1986) induced hyperlipidemia in swine that were concurrently subjected to mechanical injury by balloon abrasion of the coronary arteries. Progression of atherosclerosis over an 8-month period was compared in control animals fed a high-fat, high-cholesterol diet with that of an experimental group in which 33 ml of cod liver oil per day was added as a source of omega-3 fatty acids. The degree of hyperlipidemia in both groups of animals was comparable; concentrations of total cholesterol averaged 560 mg/dl and low-density-lipoprotein (LDL) cholesterol concentrations were 370 mg/dl. The concentration of eicosapentaenoic acid (EPA) was increased in the platelets of the cod liver oil-fed animals, and serum thromboxane B_2 concentrations were decreased. When the animals were sacrificed after 8 months on the diet, significantly less coronary artery disease was noted in the animals fed cod liver oil. The extent of luminal encroachment of atherosclerosis in the coronary arteries of the control swine was 46%, as compared to 8% in the pigs fed supplemental cod liver oil. The authors concluded that dietary cod liver oil retarded the development of coronary atherosclerosis and that this effect was possibly mediated through changes in prostaglandin metabolism.

The effect of feeding fish oil (menhaden oil) on the progression of atherosclerosis in rhesus monkeys was examined by Davis et al. (1987), and in these studies, monkeys were fed diets containing 2% cholesterol and either 25% coconut oil (group 1), 25% fish oil-coconut oil in a 1:1 mixture (group 2), or 25% fish oil-coconut oil in a 3:1 (group 3) for a period of 12 months. Serum cholesterol concentrations were significantly higher in the group 1

animals (875 mg/dl) as compared with those of group 2 (463 mg/
dl) or group 3 (405 mg/dl). When the animals were sacrificed
after 1 year on the diet, the extent of aortic intimal atherosclerosis was 79% in group 1, 48% in group 2, and 36% in group 3. The
authors concluded that replacing only 50% of the coconut oil with
fish oil reduced the serum cholesterol concentrations and inhibited
the development of atherosclerosis. However, because the serum
cholesterol levels were significantly higher in the group 1 animals,
a beneficial effect of omega-3 fatty acids over and above that attributable to reduced cholesterol levels could not be established.

In contrast to the potential beneficial effects of dietary fish
oils noted in the three previous studies, Thiery and Seidel (1987)
found an enhancement of cholesterol-induced atherosclerosis in
rabbits fed fish oils. These investigators studied three groups of
animals, the first a control group fed a cholesterol-free diet, the
second group fed an experimental diet supplemented with 1.5%
of cholesterol, and the third group receiving a similar diet to
which 2 ml day of a purified fish oil concentrate (MaxEPA) was
added. The animals remained on the diets for a period of 5
months and plasma lipids were measured throughout. The degree
of atherosclerosis was evaluated at sacrifice. Aortic atherosclerosis, determined by the extent of sudanophilic lesions, was 59%
higher in the group 3 animals fed fish oil as compared with group
2, even though serum cholesterol concentrations were similar
throughout the study period. Concentrations of serum peroxides
measured as malondialdehyde (MDA) equivalents were, however,
significantly higher in the fish oil-treated rabbits, and the authors
speculated that the enhanced atherosclerosis seen in this group
may be due to an adverse effect of oxidized lipoproteins on the
development of atherosclerosis. In light of recent data implicat-
ing a possible role for oxidized low-density lipoproteins in the
pathogenesis of atherosclerosis (Steinberg, 1987), the findings of
Thiery and Seidel warrant further investigation and underscore
that much remains to be learned concerning the health effects of
dietary supplementation with fish oil preparations in both experimental animals and humans.

No controlled trials of fish or fish oil supplementation in human subjects have been conducted in which indices of athero- sclerotic disease have been the measured end points. Thus, al- though Saynor et al. (1984) noted a significantly reduced need for sublingual nitroglycerin in a group of patients with angina pectoris who were taking 20 ml of the fish oil preparation Max- EPA per day over a 9-month period, no comparable control group was included in whom some other source of dietary fat was pro- vided.

THE EFFECTS OF DIETARY OMEGA-3 FATTY ACIDS ON PLASMA LIPIDS AND LIPOPROTEINS

Hyperlipidemia is a well-recognized risk factor for the premature development of atherosclerosis and increases in plasma cholesterol concentrations have a stronger association than does hypertrigly- ceridemia. Plasma lipids are carried as constituents of lipoprotein particles and the risks associated with increased levels of different lipoproteins differ considerably. Thus, increased plasma concen- trations of low-density lipoproteins and very-low-density-lipopro- tein (VLDL) remnants (as accumulate in the plasma of patients with type III hyperlipidemia) (Simons et al., 1987) are strongly linked to an increased risk of atherosclerosis, whereas high concen- trations of high-density lipoproteins (HDL) may afford protec- tion. Among the triglyceride-rich lipoproteins, increases in the plasma concentrations of very-low-density lipoproteins and chylo- microns do appear to be associated with an increased risk of atherosclerosis, although the data are less convincing than for pa- tients with increased plasma concentrations of VLDL remnants (Simons et al., 1987).

Numerous studies conducted over the last two decades have demonstrated that the presence of increased concentrations of omega-3 fatty acids in the diet is associated with changes in the plasma concentrations of lipids and lipoproteins. The most con- sistent finding has been a decrease in the plasma concentrations of triglycerides and VLDL particles, whereas the effects on other lipoproteins have been variable. The differences observed between different studies may be ascribed to two primary factors: first, differences in the amount of omega-3 fatty acids fed in different studies and, second, differing lipoprotein phenotypes amongst the study subjects. In this chapter we discuss selected studies in which dietary fish or fish oils rich in omega-3 fatty acids have been fed to human subjects and examine the effects of these diets on the plasma concentrations of lipids and lipoproteins in normal human subjects, patients with increased plasma concentrations of triglyceride-rich lipoproteins, and patients with primary elevations in the concentrations of LDL cholesterol. For a more detailed review, the reader is referred to the excellent report by Herold and Kinsella (1986).

STUDIES IN NORMAL HUMAN SUBJECTS

In initial studies (Harris et al., 1983), the hypolipidemic effects of diets rich in omega-6 polyunsaturated fatty acids were compared with those rich in omega-3 polyunsaturated fatty acids derived from fish and fish oils. Twelve healthy adults (six men and six women) ranging in age from 21 to 56 years participated in the outpatient study, which was carried out in a clinical research center. Three diets which differed only in fatty acid composition were fed in random order for 4 weeks each. Each diet contained 40% of calories from fat and 500 mg/day of cholesterol. The control diet contained primarily saturated fatty acids and oleic acid, and the vegetable oil-rich diet contained 54% of the total fatty acids as omega-6 polyunsaturates, whereas the diet rich in omega-3 fatty acids included long-chain omega-3 polyunsaturates fed as salmon and salmon oil. The daily intake of omega-3 fatty acids in the latter diet ranged between 20 and 29 g/day and the intake was dependent on the body weights of the study subjects. Fatty acid analysis of the plasma lipids and lipoproteins indicated that the omega-6 and omega-3 polyunsaturated fatty acids were incorporated into the cholesterol ester, phospholipid, and triglyceride components of lipoproteins, and when the subjects were on the omega-3 polyunsaturated–rich diet, the amount of arachidonic acid was reduced by 23% in the phospholipid fraction. In the 12 subjects who were fed the control diet and the salmon plus salmon oil-rich diet, total plasma cholesterol concentrations fell from 188 to 162 mg/dl ($p < 0.001$), whereas plasma triglycerides decreased from 77 to 48 mg/dl ($p < 0.005$). These changes in total plasma lipid levels were paralleled by reductions in the concentrations of VLDL cholesterol (from 13 to 8 mg/dl) and LDL cholesterol (from 128 to 108 mg/dl) on the control vs. salmon oil diet, whereas plasma concentrations of HDL remained stable (50 mg/dl on the control diet and 49 mg/dl on the salmon oil diet).

In seven subjects in whom a comparison was made between the salmon diet and the vegetable oil diet, the major difference that emerged was the unique hypotriglyceridemic effects of the diet enriched in omega-3 polyunsaturated fatty acids. Plasma concentrations of total cholesterol were 191, 170, and 174 mg/dl, respectively, on the control, salmon oil, and vegetable oil-containing diets, whereas plasma triglycerides were 76, 50, and 75 mg/dl, respectively, on the three diets. Concentrations of LDL cholesterol were reduced to a similar extent by the salmon and vegetable oils and decreased from 127 mg/dl on the control diet to 111 mg/dl on the salmon oil diet and 115 mg/dl on the vegetable oil diet. Plasma concentrations of HDL cholesterol remained stable and were not different among any of the dietary regimens. These studies indicate that large daily intakes of fish and fish oil containing 20-30 g/day of omega-3 polyunsaturated fatty acids were effective in lowering the plasma cholesterol and triglyceride concentrations, as well as the levels of VLDL and LDL, but were not found to change the levels of HDL cholesterol. Kinetic studies in which the metabolism of ^{125}I-labeled LDL was examined in control subjects fed similar amounts of omega-3 fatty acids have demonstrated that the fall in LDL cholesterol was due to a reduction in the rate of synthesis of LDL apoprotein B, whereas the fractional rate of catabolism of LDL remained unchanged (Illingworth et al., 1984).

The effects of lower doses of omega-3 fatty acids on the plasma concentrations of lipids and lipoproteins have been examined by a number of other investigators. Sanders et al (1981) evaluated the effects of a 20 ml/day supplement of cod liver oil (con-

taining 4 g/day of omega-3 fatty acids) on plasma lipids and
parameters of platelet function in 12 young men. Total cholesterol concentrations did not change significantly, whereas triglycerides fell by 23% and there was a significant increase in the plasma concentrations of HDL cholesterol. Bronsgeest-Schoute et al.
(1981) examined the effects of supplements ranging from 1.4 to
8.2 g/day of omega-3 fatty acids on plasma lipids and lipoproteins
in normal human subjects. Plasma triglyceride concentrations fell
from 90 to 55 mg/dl on the highest daily dose of omega-3 fatty
acids, but remained unchanged on doses of 1.4, 2.3, and 4.1 g/day.
Plasma concentration of total and HDL cholesterol remained unchanged on all dosages studied. Rogers et al. (1987) recently reported on a double-blind, randomized, controlled trial in which
the hypolipidemic effect of a 10-16 ml/day supplement of the
fish oil preparation MaxEPA (containing 3 g/day of omega-3 fatty
acids) was compared with a similar amount of olive oil. Concentrations of total plasma cholesterol and HDL cholesterol both rose
slightly during the trial as compared to baseline, but the change
did not reach significance. In contrast, plasma triglyceride concentrations were reduced by 54% on the fish oil supplement and increased modestly in the subjects taking olive oil.

Low-density lipoproteins are a heterogeneous group of particles of different size and potentially different degrees of athero-
genicity. Studies by Sniderman et al. (1982) have suggested that
LDL particles having a high protein-to-cholesterol ratio and a relatively high density may be particularly atherogenic. Such particles
typically are present in the plasma of patients with familial combined hyperlipidemia. The influence of a fish oil preparation containing 4 g/day of omega-3 fatty acids on LDL concentrations,
composition, and plasma concentrations of apoprotein B was
examined by Sullivan et al. (1986). Eight normal volunteers were
fed 15 ml of MaxEPA containing 4 g/day of omega-3 polyunsaturated fatty acids for a period of 2 weeks. Concentrations of total
cholesterol did not change, whereas triglycerides decreased significantly. Notably, however, plasma concentrations of LDL apoprotein B increased from 94 mg/dl at baseline to 99 mg/dl after
supplementation with the MaxEPA preparation and this increase

in LDL apoprotein B was accompanied by an increase in the protein to cholesterol ratio of isolated LDL and a decrease in mean particle diameter.

Thus, in summary, dietary supplementation with modest amounts (3-5 g/day) of omega-3 fatty acids to normal human subjects results in a significant decrease in plasma triglycerides, either no change or a modest increase in the level of HDL cholesterol, and a slight increase in the plasma concentration of LDL apoprotein B with a potential shift to a smaller, more dense LDL particle. The potential for relatively low doses of fish oils to increase plasma concentrations of LDL cholesterol and apoprotein B suggests that caution be exercised before recommending such supplements be taken by normal individuals. In contrast, when taken in larger amounts, omega-3 fatty acids cause a more profound decrease in plasma triglycerides and, concurrently, reduce the levels of LDL cholesterol. These results are consistent with the view that low doses of omega-3 fatty acids primarily reduce the synthesis of VLDL triglycerides, whereas at higher doses a concurrent reduction in the synthesis of VLDL and LDL apoprotein B also occurs.

HYPOLIPIDEMIC EFFECTS OF FISH OILS IN PATIENTS WITH HYPERTRIGLYCERIDEMIA

Increases in the plasma concentrations of triglycerides can reflect isolated elevations in the levels of VLDL (type IV phenotype), combined elevations of VLDL and LDL (type IIB phenotype), the accumulation of VLDL and potentially chylomicron remnant particles with an abnormal cholesterol enrichment in VLDL (type III hyperlipidemia), and the combined presence of increased plasma concentrations of VLDL and chylomicrons (type V phenotype). All these lipoprotein phenotypes have been associated with an increased risk of atherosclerosis, although the evidence is more controversial for those patients with only elevations in plasma triglycerides due to increased levels of VLDL particles.

The hypotriglyceridemic effects of dietary omega-3 fatty acids in patients with moderate hypertriglyceridemia due to increased plasma concentrations of VLDL particles are well estab-

lished (Herold and Kinsella, 1986). Sanders et al. (1985) studied
the effects of 15 ml/day of MaxEPA (containing 4.6 g of omega-3
fatty acids) on plasma lipids and lipoproteins in 11 patients with
primary hypertriglyceridemia. Concentrations of total cholesterol
were unaffected by the fish oil supplement, whereas triglycerides
fell from 384 to 284 mg/dl. These changes were paralleled by a
modest increase in the concentrations of HDL cholesterol (from
31 to 35 mg/dl) which was due to an increase in the HDL_3 sub-
fraction, whereas the cholesterol content of HDL_2 decreased. In
a subset of these patients, kinetic studies established that the reduction in plasma triglycerides was due to a reduced rate of synthesis of VLDL triglycerides, whereas the fractional catabolic rate
of VLDL triglycerides was not changed.

Reductions in plasma triglycerides of 25-50% have been observed by several investigators in patients with moderate hypertriglyceridemia when the intake of omega-3 polyunsaturated fatty
acids ranged from 3 to 5 g/day (Simons et al., 1985; Popp-Snijders et al., 1986; Sullivan et al., 1986). Although moderately low
doses of omega-3 fatty acids reduce VLDL cholesterol concentrations in hypertriglyceridemic subjects, the studies of Sullivan et al.
(1986) indicated that these changes could be paralleled by an increase in the plasma concentrations of LDL cholesterol and in LDL
apoprotein B. In patients with initially low levels of LDL cholesterol and concurrent hypertriglyceridemia, the LDL levels rise
into a normal range during treatment with fish oils, and this
change may not be detrimental. In contrast, in patients in whom
the LDL cholesterol concentrations increased to values above normal, the lipoprotein profile may be potentially more atherogenic
than was the case prior to fish or fish oil supplementation when
only the plasma concentrations of VLDL were increased.

In patients with combined elevations of VLDL and LDL, low
doses of omega-3 fatty acids (2.5-5 g/day) result in reduced levels
of plasma triglycerides and VLDL, but little change in total cholesterol and an increase in the plasma concentrations of LDL cholesterol (Simons et al., 1985). In previous studies, we have assessed
the hypolipidemic effects of larger amounts of omega-3 fatty acids
(30-34 g/day) in patients with combined hyperlipidemia (pheno-

typic IIB pattern), most of whom had familial combined hyperlipidemia as the genotypic reason responsible for this lipid abnormality (Phillipson et al., 1985). In 10 patients with combined elevations of VLDL and LDL studied in a metabolic ward setting, a
diet rich in fish oil at 30% of total calories lowered total plasma
cholesterol concentrations from 324 mg/dl to 236 mg/dl, whereas
triglycerides fell from 334 mg/dl at baseline to 118 mg/dl on the
fish oil diet. Plasma concentrations of VLDL cholesterol decreased substantially (from 62 mg/dl on the control diet to 17 mg/
dl on the fish oil diet), and in contrast to the effects seen at lower
doses of fish oils, plasma concentrations of LDL also fell (from
220 mg/dl on the control diet to 194 mg/dl on the fish oil-containing diet). At these doses, plasma concentrations of HDL cholesterol also fell from 41 mg/dl at baseline to 34 mg/dl on the fish
oil diet. Among the 10 subjects in this study, plasma concentrations of LDL cholesterol fell in nine and increased slightly in one.
The changes in LDL cholesterol were paralleled by decreases in
the plasma concentrations of apoprotein B, which fell from 135 to
91 mg/dl. Comparative studies in four patients who consumed
30% of total calories from fish oil during one dietary phase and
30% of their calories from vegetable oils during the second indicated that the two oils were similar in their ability to reduce
plasma concentrations of LDL cholesterol, but that the fish oil
was superior in its ability to reduce plasma triglycerides and the
concentrations of VLDL cholesterol (Phillipson et al., 1985).

Type III hyperlipoproteinemia is an uncommon disorder of
lipoprotein metabolism characterized by combined elevations of
cholesterol and triglycerides with the accumulation of cholesterol-
enriched VLDL and chylomicron remnant particles in plasma, the
development of tuberous xanthomas, and an increased risk of
coronary and peripheral vascular disease (Illingworth and Connor,
1987). Most patients with type III hyperlipoproteinemia are
homozygous for one allelic form of apoprotein E (apo E2) which
impairs the catabolism of VLDL remnant particles and, concurrently, these patients also overproduce VLDL. This combination
of an increase in VLDL production, combined with a catabolic
defect, leads to the accumulation of VLDL remnant particles

characteristic of type III hyperlipoproteinemia. Dietary omega-3
fatty acids have been demonstrated to reduce the rate of synthesis
of VLDL triglycerides and, at higher dose, to increase concurrently the fractional catabolic rate of VLDL triglycerides, reduce the
synthetic rate of VLDL apoprotein B, and reduce the synthesis of
LDL apoprotein B (Illingworth et al, 1984; Nestel et al., 1984;
Sanders et al., 1985). Dietary omega-3 fatty acids may, therefore,
have therapeutic benefit in the treatment of patients with type III
hyperlipoproteinemia. Our experience with a dietary fish oil
supplement in a 57-year-old man with type III hyperlipoproteinemia is illustrated in Figure 1. Concentrations of total cholesterol
and VLDL cholesterol decreased substantially during treatment
with 30 ml of MaxEPA per day (9 g of omega-3 fatty acids per

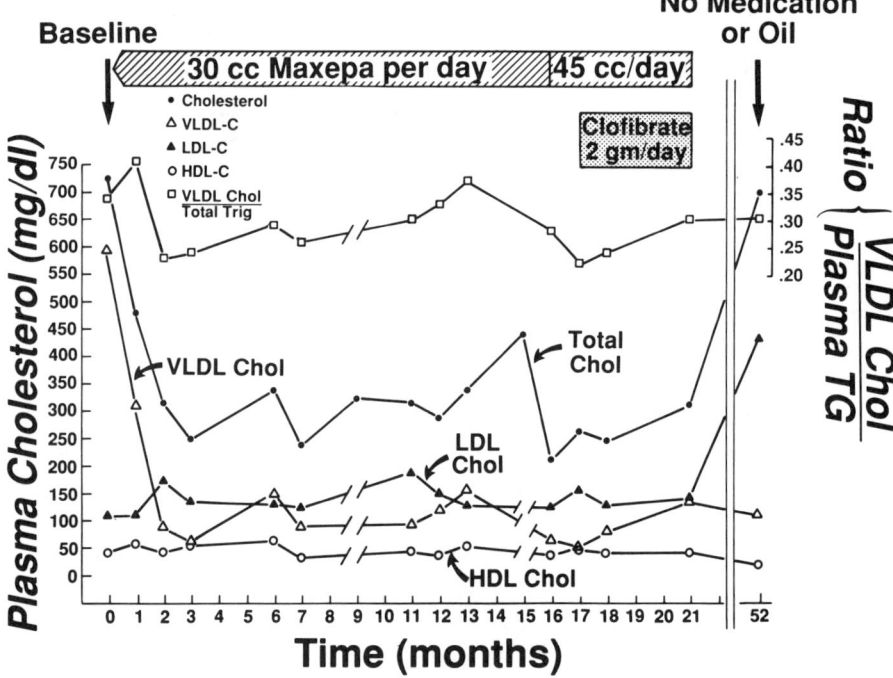

Figure 1 The effects of a dietary fish oil supplement (Max EPA)
on plasma lipids and lipoproteins in a patient with type III hyperlipoproteinemia.

day), and this effect was maintained during a prolonged period. When the dose of MaxEPA was increased to 45 ml/day, plasma concentrations of total and VLDL cholesterol fell further, but concurrent addition of clofibrate (2 g/day) resulted in no additional lipid-lowering effects. The ratio VLDL cholesterol divided by total plasma triglycerides, which is characteristically increased in patients with type III hyperlipoproteinemia, decreased during the period of fish oil treatment (Fig. 1). Upon discontinuation of the fish oil supplements, plasma lipid values rose to their original levels, indicating a lack of any prolonged carryover effect from the daily fish oil supplements. This patient had previously been treated with clofibrate and gemfibrozil as single drugs, and his response to the dietary fish oils was comparable to that seen with either lipid-lowering drug, and at a dose of 45 ml/day of MaxEPA, the result was superior. These results indicate that dietary omega-3 fatty acids may have therapeutic benefit in the treatment of patients with type III hyperlipoproteinemia who are at high risk for the premature development of atherosclerosis.

Severe hypertriglyceridemia due to the concurrent presence of chylomicron and VLDL particles, as well as chylomicron and VLDL remnants, is associated with hepatomegaly, splenomegaly, eruptive xanthomas, and the development of abdominal pain and, potentially, pancreatitis. In addition, patients with long-standing, severe hypertriglyceridemia are at an increased risk for the premature development of atherosclerosis (Zilversmit, 1979; Simons et al., 1987). In view of the unique properties of omega-3 fatty acids to reduce plasma triglyceride concentrations, one might anticipate that diets enriched in fish or fish oils would have therapeutic benefit in the treatment of patients with severe hypertriglyceridemia. Simons et al. (1985) noted reductions of 34% and 58%, respectively, in the plasma concentrations of cholesterol and triglyceride in three patients with type V hyperlipoproteinemia during the consumption of 16 g/day of a fish oil preparation containing 5 g of omega-3 fatty acids. We (Phillipson et al., 1985) have examined the comparative efficacy of fish oil and vegetable oils each fed at 20-30% of total calories as fat (20-30 g of omega-3 fatty acids or 45-60 g of omega-6 fatty acids per day, respectively) in patients with increased plasma concentrations of VLDL and chylomicrons (phenotypic type V hyperlipoproteinemia). In 10 patients studied on the control diet and then under steady-state conditions on the fish oil diet, plasma triglycerides decreased from 1353 mg/dl to 281 mg/dl, concurrently, total cholesterol concentrations decreased from 373 mg/dl to 207 mg/dl. Comparative studies on the fish oil- and vegetable oil-enriched diets were conducted in eight patients with type V hyperlipoproteinemia; the results from these studies are illustrated in Table 1. When the patients were put on the vegetable oil diet, plasma triglycerides increased rapidly, and this phase of the study was terminated after 10-14 days.

The concentrations of plasma apoproteins were determined in seven patients with type V hyperlipoproteinemia on the control diet and then, again, under steady-state conditions during con-

Table 1 The Influence of Fish and Vegetable Oils on Plasma Lipids and Lipoproteins in Patients with Type V Hyperlipoproteinemia

Diet	Lipid concentrations (mg/dl)[a]				
	Total chol.	VLDL chol.	LDL chol.	HDL chol.	TG
Control (low fat)	377 ±155	251 ±148	77 ±55	31 ± 7	1431 ±750
Fish oil (20-30% fat)	195 ± 31	74 ±67	110 ±34	35 ±12	282 ±120
Vegetable oil (20-30% fat)	264 ± 97	216 ±219	79 ±30	31 ±11	841 ±514

Data are the mean ± SD from eight patients. The fish oil diet provided 20-30 g/day of omega-3 fatty acids and the vegetable oil diet 45-60 g/day of linoleic acid.
[a]Chol. = cholesterol, TG = triglycerides.

sumption of 20-30 g/day of omega-3 fatty acids. The fish oil diet led to significant decreases in the plasma concentrations of apoproteins B, CIII, and E, and a modest decrease in the plasma concentrations of aporprotein AI (Phillipson et al., 1985).

The impressive reductions in plasma triglyceride concentrations noted in patients with phenotypic type V hyperlipoproteinemia suggest that a diet rich in fish oils and/or fish would have therapeutic benefit and that such oils can be safely incorporated into the low-fat diet recommended for use in the therapy of these patients. We have maintained several patients who had demonstrated previous intolerance to gemfibrozil or nicotinic acid on moderate doses of fish oils for 2-4 years as a therapeutic modality to reduce the risk of atherosclerosis and pancreatitis. The hypotriglyceridemic effects are maintained during such prolonged therapy.

EFFECTS OF OMEGA-3 FATTY ACIDS IN PATIENTS WITH PRIMARY HYPERCHOLESTEROLEMIA

The studies discussed in the preceding sections have indicated that consumption of fish or fish oils containing from 3 to 30 g/day of omega-3 fatty acids lowers the plasma concentrations of triglyceride-rich lipoproteins, but the effects on the concentrations of LDL cholesterol vary depending on the amount of omega-3 fatty acids consumed on a daily basis. The question, therefore, remains: Do dietary omega-3 fatty acids have any therapeutic benefit in reducing plasma concentrations of LDL cholesterol in patients with singular increases in the plasma concentrations of this lipoprotein due to primary hypercholesterolemia?

Simons et al. (1985) examined the influence of 6 and 16 ml/ day of MaxEPA on lipid and lipoprotein concentrations in nine patients with primary hypercholesterolemia who did not have concurrent hypertriglyceridemia and in whom plasma cholesterol concentrations ranged from 272 to 384 mg/dl at baseline. Although plasma triglycerides fell by a mean of 22%, there was no overall change in total plasma cholesterol concentrations. Simons et al.

concluded that at the doses employed in their studies, omega-3
fatty acids had no practical role as specific plasma cholesterol-lowering agents in patients with primary hypercholesterolemia. A
similar conclusion was reached by Brox et al. (1983), who studied
the hypolipidemic effects of a supplement of 30 ml/day of cod
liver oil (this contained 6 g of omega-3 fatty acids) in 17 adult
patients with familial hypercholesterolemia. Total plasma cholesterol concentrations were 378 mg/dl at baseline as compared to
376 mg/dl after 6 weeks on the cod liver oil supplement, whereas
LDL cholesterol concentrations were 311 mg/dl at both baseline
and 6 weeks after the cod liver oil supplement. Concentrations of
HDL cholesterol also remained stable at 49 mg/dl at baseline and
at the end of the study. Triglycerides decreased modestly in this
group of patients with initially normal triglyceride levels, and
mean values fell from 90 mg/dl at baseline to 82 mg/dl after 6
weeks on the cod liver oil supplement.

   With higher daily intakes of omega-3 fatty acids, decreases
in the plasma concentrations of total and LDL cholesterol do,
however, occur in patients with familial hypercholesterolemia.
Hatcher et al. (1987) compared the plasma lipid responses of six
patients with heterozygous familial hypercholesterolemia to two
eucaloric diets in which fat comprised 25% of total calories, with
the fish oil diet containing 20 g/day of omega-3 fatty acids. After
4 weeks on the fish oil diet, total cholesterol levels decreased from
337 to 258 mg/dl and total triglycerides fell from 138 to 63 mg/
dl. Plasma concentrations of LDL cholesterol decreased from 254
to 207 mg/dl, VLDL cholesterol fell from 26 to 13 mg/dl, and
plasma concentrations of HDL cholesterol decreased from 56 to
39 mg/dl. The fish oil diet was low in cholesterol (24 mg/1000
kcal), but in a second dietary period when additional cholesterol
was added to the fish oil-containing diet (in an amount of 200 mg/
1000 kcal/day), the hypolipidemic effects of the fish oil persisted
and concentrations of LDL cholesterol on the high cholesterol
fish oil diet rose slightly to 216 mg/dl, whereas HDL cholesterol
levels remained depressed at 38 mg/dl. These results indicate that
large daily intakes of omega-3 fatty acids lower the plasma concentrations of total, LDL, and HDL cholesterol in patients with famil-

ial hypercholesterolemia and that the fish oils blunt the anticipated rise in LDL cholesterol which would be predicted to occur
upon addition of dietary cholesterol in these patients. The latter
conclusion is similar to that of Nestel (1986), who noted that
fish oil attenuated the cholesterol-induced rise in LDL cholesterol in normal human subjects.

Optimal therapy of most adult patients with heterozygous
familial hypercholesterolemia necessitates the use of dietary measures and specific hypocholesterolemic drugs. A relevant question
to ask in terms of the therapy of these patients is, therefore, whether or not omega-3 fatty acids may have any potential to add to
the hypolipidemic effects seen with currently available drugs.
Changes in the concentrations of lipids and lipoproteins in one
adult patient with heterozygous familial hypercholesterolemia
who has been treated with lovastatin alone or in combination with
a fish oil supplement containing 11 g/day of omega-3 fatty acids
are shown in Figure 2. Concentrations of total and LDL cholesterol decreased from initial means of 404 and 331 mg/dl, respectively, at baseline to 298 and 221 mg/dl on lovastatin. During a
6-week period of fish oil supplementation, concentrations of total
and LDL cholesterol decreased from 305 and 222 mg/dl, respectively, to 268 and 194 mg/dl after 2 weeks on fish oil supplementation, decreased further to 247 and 171 mg/dl after 4 weeks, but
then total cholesterol concentrations increased to 296 mg/dl with
a rise in the LDL cholesterol to 205 mg/dl after 6 weeks on the
fish oil supplement plus lovastatin. Four weeks after discontinuation of the fish oil supplement, total cholesterol had risen to 318
mg/dl and the LDL cholesterol was 228 mg/dl. These results indicate that the addition of a fish oil preparation containing 11 g/
day of omega-3 fatty acids has a modest ability to further reduce
LDL cholesterol concentrations in a patient with familial hypercholesterolemia who remained hypercholesterolemic on single-
drug therapy with lovastatin. Plasma concentrations of HDL cholesterol in this patient were not reduced during consumption of
the fish oil supplement, whereas triglyceride levels decreased.

In conclusion, dietary omega-3 fatty acids are ineffective
as lipid-lowering agents in patients with primary hypercholestero-

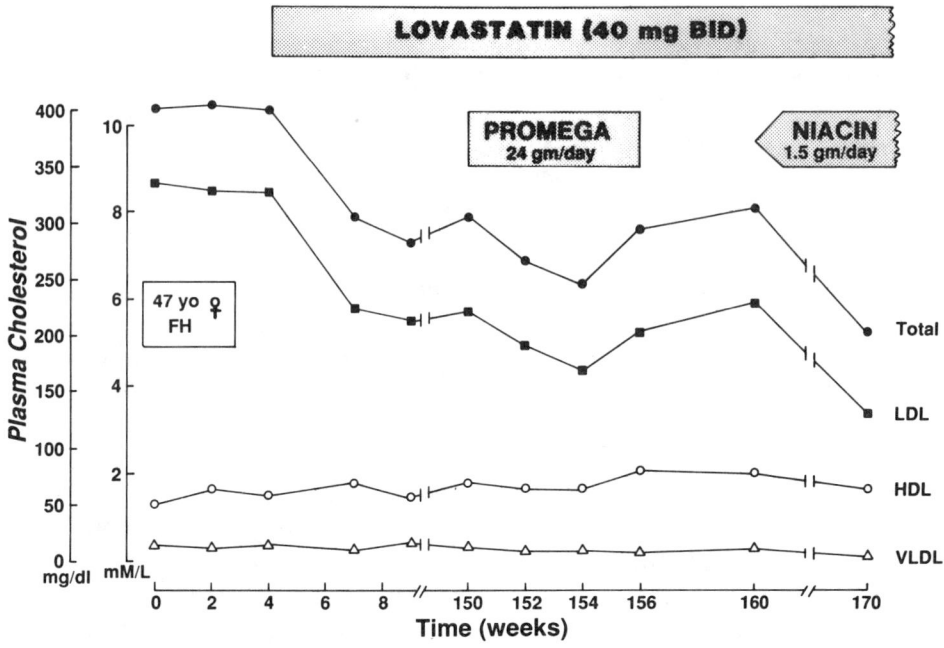

Figure 2 The influence of a fish oil supplement (Promega) containing 11 g/day of omega-3 fatty acids on plasma lipids and lipoproteins in a patient with heterozygous familial hypercholesterolemia who remained hypercholesterolemic on single-drug therapy with Lovastatin.

lemia when the doses are in the 5-6 g/day range, whereas modest decreases in plasma concentrations of both total and LDL cholesterol can be achieved with doses of approximately 20 g/day. The addition of a fish oil supplement containing 11 g/day of omega-3 fatty acids was found to have a modest LDL-lowering effect in one patient with familial hypercholesterolemia whose LDL concentrations remained high on single-drug therapy with lovastatin, but overall, omega-3 fatty acids do not appear to offer significant therapeutic benefit as LDL-lowering agents in patients with primary hypercholesterolemia.

DIETARY OMEGA-3 FATTY ACIDS AND THROMBOSIS

Abnormalities in platelet function or increased plasma concentrations of fibrinogen have been implicated as risk factors for the development of atherosclerosis. The interaction between platelets and the arterial wall is dependent on many factors, including the balance between platelet aggregation, which is promoted by increased rates of production of thromboxane A_2 in the platelet, and antiaggregatory effects of prostacyclin (PGI_2) produced by endothelial cells. The balance between these proaggregatory and antiaggregatory effects has been proposed as one factor that determines platelet reactivity, vascular tone, and potentially, release of mitogenic factors from platelets in the local environment of the arterial wall (Moncada and Vane, 1979). Epidemiological studies have established that one characteristic of Greenland Eskimos is a prolongation of bleeding time, and this has led to the speculation that part of the protective effect of dietary omega-3 fatty acids on cardiovascular disease is attributable to effects of these fatty acids on platelet function or hemostatic variables. Numerous studies, reviewed by Bradlow (1986) and Goodnight (1986), have demonstrated that dietary omega-3 fatty acids in doses of 3-5 g/day result in a prolongation in the bleeding time and, in some studies, a concurrent decrease in platelet aggregation and production of thromboxane A_2. This effect has also been observed in diabetic patients treated with 3 g/day of omega-3 fatty acids (Tilvis et al, 1987), as well as in patients with peripheral vascular disease in whom baseline rates of production of thromboxane A_2 were elevated (Knapp et al., 1986).

Despite the ability of moderate (4-6 g/day) amounts of omega-3 fatty acids to reduce parameters of platelet aggregation, concentrations of fibrinogen appear not to be affected. Haines et al. (1986) examined the effects of a 15 ml/day supplement of the fish oil preparation MaxEPA (which contains 4.5 g of omega-3 fatty acids) on blood lipids and hemostatic parameters in 41 insulin-dependent diabetics. They observed a significant reduction in thromboxane A_2 production by platelets, but an increase in fibrinogen and a concurrent increase in the plasma concentrations of LDL cholesterol. In the studies of Brox et al. (1983), in which 30 ml/day of cod liver oil was administered to 17 patients with familial hypercholesterolemia, bleeding time was not significantly prolonged, whereas collagen-induced platelet aggregation and thrombin-stimulated thromboxane A_2 production by platelets in vitro were decreased. Plasma concentrations of fibrinogen were not influenced by the fish oil supplement. Thus, moderate daily intakes of omega-3 fatty acids (3-6 g/day) appear to have favorable effects on platelet function, but do not adversely affect endothelial production of prostacyclin. However, as concluded by Knapp et al. (1986), selective inhibition of thromboxane A_2 formation may be achieved more rapidly and efficiently with low doses of aspirin. The reduced rates of development of experimental atherosclerosis in some animals fed supplemental omega-3 fatty acids (and in which concentrations of plasma lipids and lipoproteins were not different from control groups) nevertheless suggests that other properties of fish oil, such as their effects on platelet and neutrophil function, on membrane fluidity, and, perhaps, on endothelial cells, may have additional, as yet undefined, benefits in the prevention of atherosclerosis.

EFFECTS OF OMEGA-3 FATTY ACIDS ON BLOOD PRESSURE

Supplementation of the diet with fish oils or an increased intake of fish has been associated with reductions in blood pressure in several studies in normal volunteers (Hamazaki et al., 1984; Lorenz et al., 1983; Mortensen et al., 1983; Rogers et al., 1987; Sanders et al., 1981; Singer et al., 1986). In these studies, subjects were healthy normotensive male or female volunteers who ranged in age from 22 to 70 years. The lowest dose of omega-3 fatty acids studied was 1 g/day, which was consumed in canned herring by 15 subjects (Singer et al., 1986). This dose did not result in any significant decrease in systolic or diastolic blood pressure. A higher dose (4 g of omega-3 fatty acid per day) was studied by Sanders et al. (1981), and with this dose, systolic blood pressure decreased by 9 mm Hg and diastolic blood pressure fell by 10 mm

Hg. In a double-blind, crossover comparison, Mortensen et al. (1983) compared a mixture of corn oil and olive oil with a fish oil preparation containing 4 g/day of omega-3 fatty acids. Systolic blood pressure decreased by 4 mm Hg on the fish oil-containing supplement, whereas diastolic blood pressure remained unchanged. Similar results were recently obtained by Rogers et al. (1987). The highest doses of fish oil studied for their effects on blood pressure were used by Lorenz et al. (1983). These investigators studied the effects of 10 g/day of omega-3 fatty acids administered as cod liver oil over a period of 25 days; systolic blood pressure decreased by 8% and the blood pressure response to a norepinephrine infusion was also reduced, whereas no changes were noted in plasma catecholamines, renin, or urinary rates of excretion of aldosterone. The importance of studying a control group of subjects has been emphasized by the recent studies of Houwelingen et al. (1987), who compared dietary supplements of 100 g/day of mackerel or of meat on blood pressure and hematological parameters in normal volunteers. The mackerel preparation provided 4.7 g/day of omega-3 fatty acids, and dietary compliance was determined by measuring the urinary excretion of lithium which was added to both the mackerel and meat paste supplements. Systolic and diastolic blood pressures both decreased by 3-5 mm Hg on the mackerel-enriched diet, but reductions were also noted in the control group given the meat paste. When the two groups were compared, no differences in blood pressure were observed between the subjects consuming the mackerel paste and those consuming the meat paste. To what extent the reductions in blood pressure observed in both groups were due to a conditioning effect as compared to potential pharmacological effects of the dietary constitutents is unclear.

Several prospective and crossover studies have shown a modest hypotensive effect of diets enriched in omega-3 fatty acids in patients with hypertension. Rylance et al. (1986) evaluated the effects of a fish oil supplement containing 6 g/day of omega-3 fatty acids in a 3-week prospective trial in 28 adult subjects. Significant decreases in both systolic and diastolic blood pressures (19 and 8 mm Hg, respectively) were observed during the period of fish oil supplementation. Reductions in systolic blood pressure ranging from 9 to 11 mm Hg and in diastolic blood pressure ranging from 2 to 7 mm Hg have been observed in prospective or crossover trials in which supplements containing 5 g/day of omega-3 fatty acids have been fed to adult patients with mild hypertension (Singer et al,, 1985,1986). In a double-blind, crossover trial, Norris et al. (1986) examined the effects of a fish oil supplement containing 5 g/day of omega-3 fatty acids on systolic and diastolic blood pressures in 16 adults with modest hypertension (eight males, eight females). The authors observed a significant decrease in systolic blood pressure, which fell 9 mm Hg, but an insignificant reduction in the diastolic blood pressure, which decreased by 1.5 mm Hg.

Despite the lack of optimal dietary control in some of the studies cited above in which hypotensive effects have been observed with dietary supplements of 4-6 g/day of omega-3 fatty acids, the overall body of evidence favors a modest hypotensive effect of these fatty acids in normal human subjects and patients with modest hypertension. The mechanism(s) responsible for this mild hypotensive effect is largely unknown, but these changes may be related to alterations in lipid composition and/or the fluidity of cell membranes at the receptor sites for vasoactive hormones or neurotransmitters, or alternatively, local production of vasoactive prostaglandins may have a beneficial effect on the vessel wall tone and influence peripheral vascular resistance.

CLINICAL AND METABOLIC EFFECTS OF DIETARY OMEGA-3 FATTY ACIDS IN DIABETES

Patients with both type I and type II diabetes mellitus are at increased risk for the premature development of atherosclerosis. Diabetes is a risk factor for both coronary and peripheral vascular disease and several factors, including hyperglycemia, hyperaggregatory platelets, and lipoprotein abnormalities, are known to occur in the diabetic patient, all of these may be involved in the enhanced predisposition for atherosclerosis. Diabetes mellitus has been reported to be exceptionally uncommon in Greenland Eskimos, and it has been speculated that this may be linked to the dietary habits of this population. These epidemiological studies have led to several recent trials in which supplemental omega-3 fatty acids have been given to patients with either type I or type II diabetes, and the effects of these fatty acids on platelet function, lipoproteins, and parameters of glucose homeostasis have been examined.

Haines et al. (1986) examined the influence of a supplement of 15 ml/day of a fish oil supplement (MaxEPA) on blood lipids, hemostatic variables, and albuminuria in 41 patients with insulin-dependent diabetes. Thromboxane A_2 production in platelets decreased from initially elevated values; these changes were paralleled by a nonsignificant increase in bleeding time. The authors observed no change in plasma concentrations of glycosylated hemoglobin, but in assessing changes in lipids and lipoproteins, total cholesterol concentrations rose by 9%, LDL cholesterol concentrations increased by 24%, and triglycerides fell by 8%. In this study, potentially beneficial changes in platelet function appear to have been offset by potentially deleterious changes in the lipoprotein profile of the study subjects. It is interesting to note in this study that platelet aggregation and bleeding times did not change significantly, and it is possible that diabetics do not produce prostaglandin I_3 in response to fish oil supplementation in the same fashion that normal individuals do (Jones et al., 1986).

The influence of dietary omega-3 fatty acids on glycemic control and parameters of glucose homeostasis have recently been examined. Friday et al. (1987) reported on the influence of a supplement containing 8 g/day of omega-3 fatty acids on plasma lipids and glucose homeostasis in four patients with type II diabetes. Total plasma cholesterol decreased 11%, the level of VLDL cholesterol fell by 51%, and plasma triglycerides decreased by 33%. Plasma glucose levels were significantly higher in all subjects following fish oil supplementation at 30, 90, and 120 min after ingesting a mixed meal. The authors concluded that omega-3 fatty acid supplementation to this small group of subjects improved ther hypertriglyceridemia, but caused deterioration in their glycemic control. Glauber et al. (1987) examined a similar population of five type II diabetics who received a daily supplement containing 6 g/day of omega-3 fatty acids. Fasting plasma glucose concentrations rose following the fish oil supplementation, and basal hepatic glucose output also was found to increase from 2.3 to 2.9 mg/kg/min. Maximal rates of glucose disposal measured by euglycemic clamp techniques did not change significantly, and although fasting plasma insulin levels were unchanged, the mean insulin levels after a test meal were lower than was the case prior to fish oil supplementation. The authors concluded that fish oil supplementation resulted in a deterioration of diabetic control which was attributable to an increased rate of hepatic glucose output and an impaired stimulation of insulin secretion. Based on limited available data, it therefore appears that the use of omega-3 fatty acids in patients with established diabetes may favorably affect platelet function, but in certain individuals may have unfavorable effects on their plasma lipoprotein profile and potentially on their diabetic control.

The rarity of type I diabetes in Greenland Eskimos may be linked to some protective effect of their diet on the initial development of diabetes. The pathogenic process leading to islet cell loss is believed to be an autoimmune destruction of the beta cells which takes place in genetically predisposed individuals and is triggered by environmental factors. Recent evidence has strengthened the view that immunosuppressive therapy with cyclosporine can induce remission in a significant proportion of patients with newly diagnosed type I diabetes (Feutren et al. 1986). Dietary omega-3 fatty acids have been shown to change leukocyte function by reducing the production of leukotriene B_4, and it is possible that such an effect could favorably influence the early phases of islet cell destruction which occur in patients with type I diabetes.

CONCLUSIONS

The consumption of omega-3 fatty acids in the diet results in a variety of effects on lipoprotein metabolism, platelet function, and blood pressure in human subjects, the magnitude of the observed effects appears to be directly linked to the daily intake of omega-3 fatty acids. Consumption of 3-6 g/day of omega-3 fatty acids, from either fish or fish oil, lowers triglyceride concentrations and the levels of VLDL, reduces platelet production of thromboxane A_2 and may slightly prolong the Ivy bleeding time. At these doses, however, increases in plasma concentrations of LDL cholesterol and apoprotein B are observed in both normal and hypertriglyceridemic subjects and both systolic and diastolic blood pressures may decrease slightly. Based on limited information, the control of diabetes may also deteriorate owing to apparent effects of omega-3 fatty acids on hepatic glucose production and insulin secretion. Larger daily intakes of omega-3 fatty acids in the diet (15-30 g/day) exert a more profound triglyceride-lowering effect; at these doses, plasma concentrations of LDL cholesterol fall and the effects on bleeding time and thromboxane A_2 production are greater, with a significant decrease in platelet aggregation. More data are needed concerning the effects of higher doses of omega-3 fatty acids (which must be considered as equivalent to pharmaceutical treatment) on blood pressure and control of diabetes before these higher doses can be considered to have any potential therapeutic use. The major usefulness of dietary omega-3 fatty acids, therefore, is in the treatment of patients with hypertriglyceridemia, particularly those with increased plasma concentrations of chylomicrons and VLDL particles (type V hyperlipidemia), and, potentially, in the treatment of patients with type III hyperlipoproteinemia.

Studies in some animal species have indicated that dietary omega-3 fatty acids can minimize the development of atherosclerosis even when the magnitude of hypercholesterolemia in the control and experimental animals is similar. This suggests that dietary omega-3 fatty acids exert favorable effects on other factors involved in the development of atherosclerosis; these may include effects on platelet function, leukotriene B_4 production, or direct effects on the arterial wall. Although dietary omega-3 fatty acids may favorably affect some cardiovascular risk factors, they may have adverse effects on others; for this reason, the use of supplemental fish oils cannot be generally recommended. Although epidemiological studies have indicated a lower incidence of cardiovascular disease in populations with a high habitual intake of fish, it is unclear to what extent this apparent protection is due to the presence of omega-3 fatty acids in the fish, as compared to other components, or to the fact that most of these subjects are consuming lower amounts of saturated fatty acids in their diets.

Further studies are needed to define the potential beneficial roles of individual long-chain omega-3 fatty acids (EPA as compared to DHA) on lipoprotein metabolism, platelet function, and other cardiovascular risk factors in human subjects, as well as to define better the dose-response relationship between daily intake of these fatty acids and their effects on plasma lipoproteins, platelet function, and prostaglandin metabolism.

ACKNOWLEDGMENTS

This work was supported in part by Research Grants HL28399, HL37940, the General Clinical Research Center's Program (RR-334), National Institutes of Health, and by the American Heart Association, Oregon Affiliate.

REFERENCES

Bang HO, Dyerberg J, Hjrne NA. Composition of food consumed by Greenland Eskimos. Acta Med Scand 1976,200:69-73.

Bradlow BA. Thrombosis and omega-3 fatty acids. Epidemiological and clinical aspects. In: Simopoulas AP, Kifer RR, Martin RE, eds. Health effects of polyunsaturated fatty acids in seafoods. New York, Academic Press, 1986; 111-133.

Bronsgeest-Schoute HC, Van Gent CM, Luten JB, Ruiter A. The effect of various intakes of omega-3 fatty acids on the blood lipid composition in healthy human subjects. Am J Clin Nutr 1981,34:1752-1757.

Brox JH, Killie JE, Osterud B, et al. Effects of cod liver oil on platelets and coagulation in familial hypercholesterolemia. Acta Med Scand 1983;213:137-144.

Casali RE, Hale JA, Lenerz L, et al. Improved graft patency associated with altered platelet function induced by marine fatty acids in dogs. J Surg Res 1986;40:6-12.

Davis HR, Bridenstine RT, Vesselinovitch D, Wissler, RW. Fish oil inhibits the development of atherosclerosis in rhesus monkeys. Arteriosclerosis 1987;7:441-447.

Feutren G, Assan R, Karsenty G, et al. Cyclosporine increases the rate and length of remissions in insulin dependent diabetes of recent onset. Lancet 1986;2:119-123.

Friday KE, Childs M, Fujimoto W, et al. The effect of omega-3 fatty acid supplementation on glucose hemostasis and plasma lipoproteins in type II diabetic subjects. Clin Res 1987;35:193A.

Glauber HS, Wallace P, Brechtel G. Adverse effects of omega-3 fatty acids on non-insulin dependent diabetes mellitus. Clin Res 1987;35:504A.

Goodnight SH, Jr. The antithrombotic effects of fish oil. In: Simopoulas AP, Kifer RR, Martine RE, eds. Health effects of polyunsaturated fatty acids in seafoods. New York: Academic Press, 1986, 135-149.

Haines AP, Sanders TAB, Imeson JD, et al. Effects of a fish oil supplement on platelet function, hemostatic variables and albuminuria in insulin dependent diabetics. Thrombosis Res 1986,43:643-655.

Hamazaki T, Nakazawa R, Tateno S, et al. Effects of fish oil rich in eicosapentaenoic acid on serum lipid in hyperlipidemic hemodialysis patients. Kidney Int 1984,26:81-84.

Harris WS, Connor WE, McMurry MP. The comparative reduction of the plasma lipids and lipoproteins by dietary polyunsaturated fats: salmon oil vs. vegetable oils. Metabolism 1983;32:179-184.

Hatcher LF, Connor WE, Ullmann DO, et al. Dietary fish oil in

familial hypercholesterolemia: response to added cholesterol. Clin Res 1987,35:772A.

Herold PM, Kinesella JE. Fish oil consumption and decreased
risk of cardiovascular disease: a comparison of findings from
animal and human feeding trials. Am J Clin Nutr 1986;43:
566-598.

Houwelingen RV, Nordoy A, Vanderbeek E, et al. Effect of a
moderate fish intake on blood pressure, bleeding time, hema-
tology and clinical chemistry in healthy males. Am J Clin
Nutr 1987,46:424-436.

Illingworth DR, Connor WE. Disorders of lipid metabolism. In:
Felig P, Baxter JD, Broadus AE, Frohman LA, eds. Endocrinology and metabolism. New York: McGraw-Hill, 1987:
1244-1314.

Illingworth DR, Harris WS, Connor WE. Inhibition of low density
lipoprotein synthesis by dietary omega-3 fatty acids in humans. Arteriosclerosis 1984;4:270-275.

Jones DB, Haitas B, Bound EG, et al. Platelet aggregation in non-
insulin dependent diabetes: association with platelet fatty
acids. Diabetic Med 1986;3:52-55.

Kagawa Y, Nishizawa M, Suzuki M, et al. Eicosapentaenoic acid
of serum lipids of Japanese islanders with low incidence of
cardiovascular diseases. J Nutr Sci Vitaminol 1982;28:441-
453.

Knapp HR, Reilly IAG, Alessandrini P, Fitzgerald GA. In vivo in-
dexes of platelet and vascular function during fish-oil administration in patients with atherosclerosis. N Engl J Med 1986;
314:937-942.

Kromhout D, Bosschieter EB, Coulander C. The inverse relation
between fish comsumption and 20-year mortality from coronary heart disease. N Engl J Med 1985,312:1205-1209.

Lorenz R, Spengler U, Fischer S, et al. Platelet function, thromboxane formation and blood pressure control during supplementation of the Western diet with cod liver oil. Circulation
1983,67:504-511.

Moncada S, Vane JR. Arachidonic acid metabolites and the inter-actions between platelets and blood vessel walls. N Engl J Med 1979,300:1142-1147.

Mortensen JZ, Schmidt EB, Nielsen AH, Dyerberg J. The effect of omega-6 and omega-3 polyunsaturated fatty acids on hemostasis, blood lipids and blood pressure. Thromb Haemost 1983;50:543-546.

Nestel PJ. Fish oil attenuates the cholesterol induced rise in lipoprotein cholesterol. Am J Clin Nutr 1986;43:752-757.

Nestel PJ, Connor WE, Reardon MR, et al. Suppression by diets rich in fish oil of very low density lipoprotein production in man. J Clin Invest 1984,74:82-89.

Norris PG, Jones CJ, Weston MJ. Effect of dietary supplementa-tion with fish oil on systolic blood pressure in mild essential hypertension. Br Med J 1986,293:104-105.

Phillipson BE, Rothrock DW, Connor WE, et al. Reduction of plasma lipids lipoproteins and apoproteins by dietary fish oil in patients with hypertriglyceridemia. N Engl J Med 1985;312:1210-1216.

Popp-Snijders C, Schouten JA, Heine RJ, Vanderven EA. Dietary omega-3 polyunsaturated fatty acids lower plasma triacyl-glycerol concentrations in noninsulin dependent diabetes mellitus. Atherosclerosis 1986;61:253-254.

Rogers S, James KS, Butland BK, et al. Effects of a fish oil sup-plement on serum lipids, blood pressure, bleeding time, he-mostatic and rheological variables. A double blind random-ized controlled trial in healthy volunteers. Atherosclerosis 1987,63:137-143.

Ross R. The pathogenesis of atherosclerosis: an update. N Engl J Med 1986,314:488-500.

Rylance PB, Gordge MP, Saynor R, et al. Fish oil modifies lipids and reduces platelet aggregability in hemodialysis patients. Nephron 1986;43:196-202.

Sanders TAB, Vickers M, Haines AP. Effect on blood lipids and hemostasis of a supplement of cod-liver oil, rich in eicosapen-

taenoic and docosahexaenoic acids, in healthy young men.
Clin Sci 1981;61:317-324.

Sanders TAB, Sullivan DR, Reeve J, Thompson GR. Triglyceride
lowering effect of marine polyunsaturates in patients with
hypertriglyceridemia. Arteriosclerosis 1985;5:459-465.

Saynor R, Verel D, Gillott T. The long term effects of dietary
supplementation with fish lipid concentrate on serum lipids,
bleeding time, platelets and angina. Atherosclerosis 1984;50:
3-10.

Simons LA, Hickie JB, Balasubramaniam S. On the effects of
omega-3 fatty acids (MaxEPA) on plasma lipids and lipoproteins in patients with hyperlipidemia. Atherosclerosis 1985;
54:75-88.

Simons LA, Dwyer T, Simons J, et al. Chylomicrons and chylomicron remnants in coronary artery disease. A case control
study. Atherosclerosis 1987;65:181-189.

Singer P, Wirth M, Godicke W, Heine H. Blood pressure lowering
effect of eicosapentaenoic acid-rich diet in normotensive,
hypertensive and hyperlipidemic subjects. Experientia 1985;
41.462-464.

Singer P, Berger I, Wirth M, et al. Slow desaturation and elongation of linoleic and alpha linolenic acids as a rationale of eicosapentaenoic acid-rich diet to lower blood pressure and serum
lipids in normal, hypertensive and hyperlipidemic subjects.
Prostaglandins Leukotriens Med 1986;24:173-193.

Sniderman AD, Wolfson C, Tang B, et al. Association of hyper-
apobetalipoproteinemia with endogeneous hypertriglyceridemia and atherosclerosis. Ann Intern Med 1982;97:833-
839.

Steinberg D. Lipoproteins and the pathogenesis of atherosclerosis.
Circulation 1987,76:508-514.

Sullivan DR, Sanders TAB, Trayner IM, Thompson GR. Paradoxi-
cal elevation of LDL and apoprotein B levels in hypertriglyceridemic patients and normal subjects ingesting fish oil.
Atherosclerosis 1986,61:129-134.

Thiery J, Seidel D. Fish oil feeding results in an enhancement of cholesterol induced atherosclerosis in rabbits. Atherosclerosis 1987;63:53-56.

Tilvis RS, Rasi V, Viinikka L, et al. Effects of purified fish oil on platelet lipids and function in diabetic women. Clin Chim Acta 1987;164:315-322.

Weiner BH, Ockene IS, Levine PH, et al. Inhibition of atherosclerosis by cod liver oil in a hyperlipidemic swine model. N Engl J Med 1986,315:841-846.

Zilversmit DB. Atherogenesis: a postprandial phenomenon. Circulation 1979,60:473-479.

3
Clinical and Epidemiological Data on the Effects of Fish Oil in Cardiovascular Disease

Charles H. Hennekens, Julie E. Buring, and Sherry L. Mayrent
Harvard Medical School and Brigham and Women's Hospital
Boston, Massachusetts

I. INTRODUCTION

Most epidemiological hypotheses are formulated from either astute clinical observations or descriptive epidemiological studies, which compare the overall experience observed for a population with an expected value. Once the hypothesis is formulated, subsequent evaluation generally evolves along two fronts, often simultaneously. First, basic researchers attempt to identify possible mechanisms to explain why an exposure causes or prevents disease. Second, by collecting information on the previous health habits and exposures of individuals in case-control studies or observing the subsequent health experiences of those with and without a particular exposure in cohort studies, epidemiologists attempt to determine whether an exposure causes or prevents disease. In addition, to evelute the small to moderate effects that are most plausible, but nonetheless clinically important, ideally randomized trials are conducted, if not precluded by ethical, cost, or feasibility considerations (Hennekens and Buring, 1987).

This framework is useful in considering the current state of knowledge concerning fish oil and cardiovascular disease. The hypothesis that marine oils may prevent cardiovascular disease was formulated from descriptive epidemiological data, primarily among Eskimos in Greenland. In this population, cardiovascular disease is extremely rare and the usual diet consists almost exclusively of marine mammals and fish. Subsequent investigations have concentrated on the identification of possible mechanisms, focusing specifically on the effects of omega-3 fatty acids on cardiovascular risk factors rather than on cardiovascular disease itself (Illingworth, 1987). This chapter summarizes the available epidemiological data and outlines the priorities for future research upon which public policy could be based.

THE POTENTIAL PUBLIC HEALTH IMPACT OF FISH OIL IN THE UNITED STATES

The importance of the potential effect of fish oil relates to the public health impact of cardiovascular disease in the United States and other developed nations. In the United States alone, there are more than 2 million deaths annually. The single leading cause of these deaths is coronary heart disease, which accounts for 34% of all fatalities. Stroke accounts for another 7% of deaths, so that total cardiovascular disease causes about 41%, or more than 800,000 annual U.S. deaths (US DHHS, 1985).

The major independent risk factors for coronary heart disease are cigarette smoking, blood pressure level, and level of blood cholesterol. With respect to cigarettes, current smokers have about a 60-80% increased risk of death from CHD (US DHHS, 1983; Hennekens and Buring, 1985). As regards level of blood pressure, in an overview of randomized trials of pharmacological therapy for mild to moderate hypertension (Hebert et al., 1988), a decrease in diastolic blood pressure of 8 mm Hg corresponded to an approximate 40% decrease in risk of fatal and nonfatal stroke and a 12% decrease in risk of coronary heart disease. The public health benefit of cholesterol lowering derives from basic research as well as both observational and experimental epidemiological studies. In an overview of 19 trials of this intervention (Consensus Conference, 1985), for a 10% reduction in cholesterol, there was a corresponding 12% reduction in risk of cardiac death, a 30% reduction in risk of nonfatal myocardial infarction, and a 20% reduction in the risk of experiencing a first cardiac event.

These risk reductions are small to moderate, but for a disease as common as coronary heart disease, even a small reduction in risk of 10-30% will affect very large numbers of individuals. Specifically, if decreasing blood pressure or, more likely, cholesterol level with fish oil caused a net reduction in risk of death from coronary heart disease of even 20%, a large-scale intervention program could, at least in theory, prevent over 100,000 premature deaths from coronary disease each year in the United States alone.

DESCRIPTIVE STUDIES OF MARINE-BASED DIETS AND CORONARY HEART DISEASE

While the effects of omega-3 fatty acids on lipids have been the subject of research for many years (Stansby, 1969), specific interest in their possible preventive role in coronary heart disease (CHD) was stimulated by the results from a number of studies of the Eskimos of Northwest Greenland (Eskimo diets, 1983). Specifically, among a population of approximately 1800 Greenland Eskimos, only three cases of myocardial infarction occurred over a 25-year follow-up period, while 40 such cases would have been expected on the basis of disease rates in Denmark, the nearest and presumably most comparable European country (Kromann and Green, 1980).

In investigating possible reasons for this low incidence of CHD, Bang and colleagues (Bang et al., 1971) found that Greenland Eskimos had a more favorable lipid profile than Danes. Specifically, as shown in Table 1, the mean total cholesterol value among the male Eskimos was 233 mg/100 ml, compared with 273 mg/100 ml among the Danish men, and mean triglycer-

Table 1 Total Cholesterol and Triglyceride Levels in Greenland
Eskimos and Danish Men

	Mean values (mg/100 ml)[a]	
	Eskimos	Danes
Total cholesterol	233	273
Triglycerides	57	129

[a]For both differences, $p < 0.001$.

ide levels were 57 and 129 mg/100 ml, respectively. Both these
differences were statistically significant. A similar pattern was
found for low-density-lipoprotein (LDL) cholesterol and very-low-
density-lipoprotein (VLDL) cholesterol. The corresponding values
for women were similar. In addition, male Eskimos had significantly higher levels of high-density-lipoprotein (HDL) cholesterol,
increased levels of which have been associated with decreased risk
of CHD. There were, however, no significant differences in HDL
cholesterol between female Eskimos and Danes. In this study,
lipid levels in the Danish group increased with age, the pattern
common in developed countries, while among the Eskimos lipid
values remained fairly constant. Thus, the differences in lipid
values between the two populations increase with age and become
even more pronounced in the older age groups, who are at higher
risks for developing CHD.

Dietary Fats, Lipids, and Coronary Heart Disease

The lipid pattern observed in this Eskimo population is consistent
with established knowledge of decreased risks of CHD associated
with low levels of total cholesterol, triglycerides, LDL, and VLDL
and higher levels of HDL cholesterol (Wallace and Anderson,
1987). However, this type of favorable blood lipid profile is most
commonly associated with low intakes of dietary fat, as in a developed country like Japan or a developing country such as the
People's Republic of China. In fact, the percentage of total calor-

Table 2   Percentages of Total Fatty Acids by Types of Dietary
Fat in Eskimo and Danish Diets

Type of fat	% total fatty acids	
	Eskimos	Danes
Saturated	22.8	52.7
Monounsaturated	57.3	34.6
Polyunsaturated	19.2	12.7
P/S ratio	0.8	0.2

ies obtained from fats in the average Eskimo diet is virtually iden-
cal to that of the diet in Denmark, where risks of CHD are much
higher, being 39% and 42%, respectively (Bang et al., 1980).
Moreover, the Eskimos obtained nearly twice as many of their
total calories from protein as did the Danes. Since the main Eskimo food sources are marine mammals and fish (Bang et al., 1976),
it appeared that their diet might be even higher in cholesterol than
the European diet. Indeed, when the specific intake was measured, it turned out that the average daily intake of cholesterol
was 245 mg/1000 cal for the Eskimos, compared with only 139
among the Danes. However, as shown in Table 2, the Eskimos
consume a markedly lower proportion of saturated fats, which are
associated with increased cholesterol levels, and a higher proportion of cholesterol-lowering polyunsaturates. Their P/S ratio,
which is inversely related to coronary risk, is also much higher
than that of the Danes (Bang et al., 1980).

Additional blood analyses indicated that compared with the
Danish group, the Eskimos had lower concentrations of lineoleic
or omega-6 fatty acids and higher concentrations of linolenic or
omega-3 fatty acids, especially the long-chain polyunsaturated
fatty acids, eicosapentaenoic (EPA) and docosahexaenoic (Bang
et al., 1980). The most marked differences were in linoleic acid
levels, which were 10.0 g/day/3000 kcal in the Danes compared
with 5.4 g/day in the Eskimos, and levels of EPA, which consti-
tuted up to 4.6% of total fatty acids in Eskimos but only 0.5%
in Danes (Bang et al., 1980). Thus, it appears that in Eskimos,

the polyunsaturated fatty acids of the omega-6 family, such as linoleic acid, which predominate in developed countries, are replaced by those of the omega-3 family, such as EPA. This pattern reflects the predominance in their diet of marine mammals and cold-water fish, which have a relatively high total fat content composed primarily of these particular fatty acids.

Fish Oils and Platelet Function

Although lower levels of triglycerides and LDL and VLDL cholesterol and higher levels of HDL cholesterol may, in part, explain the lower incidence of CHD among Greenland Eskimos, an increased bleeding tendency has also been observed in this population. This suggests that decreased platelet aggregability may also contribute to their lower risk of CHD. Comparison of bleeding times between 21 Greenland Eskimos and 21 age- and sex-matched Danish controls (Dyerberg and Bang, 1979) revealed marked differences in this value, with a mean of 8.05 min in Eskimos and 4.76 min in Danes. Moreover, the second phase of platelet aggregation occurred in only 48% of specimens from Eskimo subjects, while secondary-phase aggregation was achieved in all plasma samples of Danish participants. Finally, the mean platelet count was 171,000/ml among Eskimos, compared with 232,000 among Danes. The investigators suggested that omega-3 fatty acids influence the synthesis of prostaglandins that regulate platelet aggregation. While the substrate for prostaglandin synthesis in Danes is exclusively arachidonic acid, in Eskimos it also includes omega-3 fatty acids, and this makeup may favor the production of antiaggregatory prostacycline over that of proaggregatory prostaglandins.

Other Descriptive Data

Similar observations have been reported among Indians on Vancouver Island (Bates et al., 1985), who eat a diet chiefly composed of salmon, as well as among Japanese living in fishing villages (Hirai et al., 1980; Kagawa et al., 1982). Both groups have significantly lower blood cholesterol levels than their non-fish-eating counterparts, and the Japanese also have been reported to have increased bleeding times (Hirai et al., 1980).

Nature or Nurture?

Before considering whether omega-3 intake itself decreases the incidence of CHD in these populations, it is first necessary to address the possibility that there are genetic differences, rather than dietary differences, between the groups who do and do not consume high-fish diets that could account for the effects on lipids and platelets. This possibility has been examined in migrant studies, a type of investigation in which the experience of a particular racial or ethnic group in its native environment is compared with that of members of that group who have migrated to a geographical area with a different lifestyle to determine whether the migrants more closely resemble the population they came from or the host population (Hennekens and Buring, 1987). This point can be illustrated using data from the studies among Greenland Eskimos. As shown in Table 3, when the lipid profiles of female Eskimos who had migrated to Denmark were compared with those of both female Eskimos living in Greenland and native Danish women, the lipid profiles of the migrant Eskimos were found to resemble those of the Danish women more closely than

Table 3   Total Cholesterol and Triglyceride Levels in Greenalnd Eskimo Women, Migrant Eskimo Women in Denmark, and Native Danish Women

	Mean lipids (mg/100 ml)		
	Eskimos in Greenland	Eskimos in Denmark	Danish women
Total cholesterol	218	286	264
Triglycerides	43	112	98

those of Greenland Eskimos (Bang and Dyerberg, 1972). In each instance, the values among the migrants were significantly different from those of the Greenland Eskimos and not significantly different from those of the Danes. These data indicate that genetic factors are not chiefly responsible for the more favorable lipid profiles found among Greenland Eskimos.

ANALYTICAL STUDIES OF FISH OIL AND CORONARY HEART DISEASE

While all these descriptive data are intriguing, it is important to bear in mind that it is not possible to use such information to test the hypothesis that a high intake of omegea-3 fatty acids is associated with a decreased risk of cardiovascular disease. To do so requires the conduct of analytical epidemiological studies designed to address this question specifically. Unfortunately, very little analytical epidemiological data are available concerning the incidence of cardiovascular disease in relation to consumption of fish or other foods containing the omega-3-rich, polyunsaturated fatty acids.

Perhaps the major observational analytical study of this question is the Zutphen study (Kromhout et al., 1985), which gathered data in 1960 on fish consumption from 852 middle-aged Dutch men with no history of CHD and followed them for 20 years. As shown in Table 4, for each level of fish intake, there was a marked reduction in risk of fatal CHD, which was of borderline statistical significance. Overall, there was a statistically significant inverse trend of increasing level of fish consumption with decreased risk of CHD. Those in the highest intake group had a nearly 60% reduction in risk of mortality from CHD compared with those who ate no fish at all, and even those in the lowest intake groups experienced a 40% reduction. Interestingly, this study showed no relationship of fish consumption with the major risk factors, including age, total cholesterol level, blood pressure, and cigarette smoking. The authors concluded that eating as few as two fish meals per week could result in a reduction of risk of death from coronary heart disease. This conclusion is of particu-

Table 4 Zutphen Study of Fish Consumption and CHD Risk in Men

Fish consumption (g/day)	RR of CHD death	95% CL
0	1.00	—
1-14	0.60	0.33-1.10
15-29	0.57	0.30-1.09
30-44	0.46	0.20-1.06
45+	0.42	0.16-1.13

p value for trend <0.05.

lar note because an average fish intake of two meals per week is roughly 20g/day, compared with 400 g average daily consumption among the Greenland Eskimos (Bang and Dyerberg, 1972).

These intriguing results have been widely cited as indicating the value of consuming small amounts of fish as a means of reducing risk of coronary heart disease. However, a number of problems or limitations should be considered before such a conclusion can be drawn. First, while the investigators controlled for a large number of cardiovascular risk factors, they did not have available information on either lipoprotein subfractions or triglycerides, the components of blood cholesterol most likely to be affected by dietary EPA. The fact that the EPA content of the average fish diet consumed by these Dutch men is very low supports the possibility that some unidentified confounding factor is responsible, at least in part, for the observed results. It may be some component of the fish, other than omega-3 fatty acids, or even some other lifestyle factor practiced or avoided by those who consume fish, that accounts for the risk reductions observed in this study.

The reported findings from the Zutphen study prompted investigators in the Western Electric Study (Shekelle et al., 1985) to examine these questions in their data on nearly 2000 men in Chicago who were free from CHD in 1957 and had been followed for 25 years. As shown in Table 5, the results of this analysis were

Table 5 Western Electric Study of Fish Consumption and CHD Risk in Men

Fish consumption (g/day)	RR of CHD death
0	1.00
1-17	0.91
18-34	0.76
35+	0.63

p value for trend = 0.008.

similar, with a statistically significant inverse association of fish consumption with CHD risk. This relationship persisted after controlling for the major CHD risk factors as well as percentage of calories from polyunsaturated fats, total calories, and alcohol intake.

In contrast, two other reports, also prompted by the publication of the Zutphen study, did not corroborate these findings. The first (Vollset et al., 1985) compared observed and expected deaths from CHD by frequency of fish consumption among 11,000 Norwegian men followed from 1968 to 1981. Table 6 shows that there were no significant differences either for total CHD deaths or for deaths from acute myocardial infarction (MI)

Table 6 Norwegian Study of Fish Consumption and CHD Risk in Men

Fish meals per month	CHD Deaths		Fatal 1st MI	
	Obs	Exp	Obs	Exp
0-4	49	55.4	17	18.2
5-14	596	592.3	185	188.9
15-24	284	278.7	83	82.2
25+	38	40.7	16	11.6

Obs = observed; Exp = expected.

Table 7 Japanese Study of Fish Consumption and CHD Risk in Men

Frequency of fish intake	RR of CHD death
Almost never	1.00
<2/week	1.86
2-4/week	1.76
Almost daily	1.66

among the subgroup of men with no previous history of cardio-vascular disease. The second study shown in Table 7, was conducted among 7615 Japanese men with no history of coronary disease as part of the Honolulu Heart Program (Curb and Reed, 1985). After 12 years of follow-up, the age-adjusted relative risks of CHD death were actually higher overall among those consuming fish regularly, although there was a suggestion of decreasing trend among the three highest fish consumption categories. This situation may have resulted from the very small number of men in the "almost never" category of fish consumption. Similar results were obtained when CHD rates were compared according to amount of fish consumed during the 24 h prior to the baseline interview as assessed by dietary recall.

In evaluating these observational analytical studies, it is important to bear in mind that the exposure measured was total consumption, of which fish high in EPA may be only a small proportion. For example, only one-third of the fish consumed by the Dutch population fell into the category rich in omega-3 fatty acids. This raises the question of whether the EPA in high-fish diets contributes to decreased risks of CHD.

CURRENT STATUS OF KNOWLEDGE AND FUTURE PERSPECTIVES

Thus, with respect to the relationship of consumption of marine oils with risk of cardiovascular disease, there is a large body of

evidence indicating that intake of omega-3 fatty acids favorably
alters lipid profiles, decreases platelet function, and may decrease
blood pressure. However, we do not yet know whether altering
these risk factors will lead to a favorable risk-to-benefit ratio for
cardiovascular disease itself. Second, descriptive data from Greenland Eskimos, Kitasoo Indians, and Okinawan Japanese all suggest
that their low incidence of CHD results from diets rich in omega-3.
However, while such descriptive studies are extremely useful for
the formulation of hypotheses, they cannot adequately be tested.
Finally, some, but not all, observational studies indicate that individuals who consume higher than average amounts of fish may
have a decreased risk of death from coronary heart disease. In
addition to the lack of consistency of these findings, it is also not
possible to determine whether any observed effect is due to the
omega-3 fatty acid content of the fish consumed. The question
then remains, where do we go from here?

The ultimate goal of any further research in this area is to
enable us to make an informed decision concerning both public
policy and clinical practice. Clinicians need to know how to ad-
vise patients, particularly with respect to evaluating the large numbers of products currently and increasingly being advertised as
ways to avoid coronary heart disease. The general public needs
to know whether there are safe, practicable changes in or addi-
tions to our diets that we can implement in order to reduce the
risk of developing coronary disease. Given the current state of
knowledge, the best and possibly only way to answer these questions definitively is to conduct large-scale, randomized trials.

Such trials should be very large, to achieve adequate statistical power to detect the small to moderate risk reductions that
are most likely. In addition, it is essential that they assess the
effects of fish oils on the actual end points of interest—namely
incidence of CHD death and perhaps nonfatal MI—rather than
on the risk factors for those end points, such as cholesterol level
or blood pressure. Finally, because the end points of greatest
interest are chronic diseases with long latency periods. It is important that any trial of fish oil allow sufficient follow-up time
for the intervention to have an effect. If the mechanism of effect

is through a decrease in platelet function, which occurs almost immediately, a shorter follow-up period might be sufficient, while if, as is perhaps more likely, the mechanism by which omega-3 fatty acids reduce CHD is through an effect on lipids, longer durations of follow-up would be necessary.

It will also be essential to evaluate the possible side effects of the intervention in relation to possible benefits for primary prevention as well as secondary prevention or therapy. In therapeutic situations where people already have the disease in question, such as MI, or even in circumstances in which an intervention is targeted to individuals identified as being at particularly high risk of developing the disease, such as patients with hyperlipidemia, higher levels of discomfort, inconvenience, or even risks of developing associated conditions may be tolerable. Among previously healthy people at usual risk, however, even slight elevations in frequency of unpleasant or deleterious side effects may well be more than either can or should be tolerated.

In the case of marine oils, these needs are particularly pressing. In the Eskimo and Indian populations described earlier, the low levels of arachidonic acid, a precursor of thromboxane A_2 which has a strong effect on both thrombotic and vasodilatory processes, suggests that these two populations have, perhaps through evolution, developed mechanisms for ensuring adequate hemostasis (Bates et al., 1985). In Europeans, however, a lack of such mechanisms could make drastic dietary changes, through either consumption of large amounts of fish or addition of fish oil capsules, a particular hazard. Any trial of such an intervention would have to monitor platelet function and bleeding time very carefully to be able to determine whether there is a net benefit of the intervention. In fact, since fish oil has pharmacological effects similar to those of aspirin, it would be necessary to monitor participants closely for the deleterious effects that have been reported in trials of antiplatelet therapy, which include increased risks of both gastric and cerebral hemorrhage (Anti-Platelet Trialists Collaboration, 1987).

Finally, if such trials are conducted, they should be done very soon. The timing of any randomized trial is a particularly delicate matter. For both ethical and practical reasons, there must be sufficient doubt generally about the intervention to be tested to allow withholding it from half the participants, at the same time as there must be sufficient belief in its potential to justify exposing the other half (Hennekens and Buring, 1987). In the case of fish oil, claims of the beneficial effects of various preparations can be found in health food stores as well as newspapers and magazines all over the United States. Each new report of a small, short-term study of fish oil is likely to increase this advertising, and consequent sales even further. One fear is that use of these products will continue to increase even in the absence of reliable evidence derived from large, well-designed studies in humans. Even if such trials were to show a net benefit, it would be unfortunate for a middle-aged hyperlipidemic or hypertensive person or cigarette smoker to take a fish oil capsule to reduce risks of vascular mortality. On the other hand, if there is truly no material reduction in total cardiovascular death rates among people who consume fish oil in foods or supplements, then the widespread prophylactic use of marine oils might even do more harm, die to increased bleeding, than good. Such trials would also need to address the question of minimum effective dose and optimal duration of treatment.

CONCLUSION

In conclusion, with respect to the hypothesis that fish oil reduces risk of cardiovascular disease, the available data are intriguing and exciting, but far from conclusive. The major gap in knowledge at this time seems to be whether high intake of marine oils reduces risk of developing a myocardial infarction or death due to cardiovascular disease. In that regard, it may be particularly worthwhile to conduct randomized trials that are well designed and of adequate size to answer this question definitively, either by proving that supplementing the diet with omega-3 fatty acids reduces these risks, or by establishing reliably that this intervention is ineffective. If and when sound data become available from such trials, it will be possible to develop public policy concerning fish oils. Until that time, the general public should be advised to continue intervention strategies, such as cholesterol lowering, for which the risks and benefits are already known and quantified.

REFERENCES

Anti-Platelet Trialists Collaboration (Barnett H, Bousser et al.). Secondary prevention of vascular disease by prolonged antiplatelet therapy. Br Med J 1988;296:320-331.

Bang HO, Dyerberg J. Plasma lipids and lipoproteins in Greenlandic West Coast Eskimos. Acta Med Scand 1972;192: 85-94.

Bang HO, Dyerberg J, Nielsen AB. Plasma lipid and lipoprotein pattern in Greenlandic West-Coast Eskimos. Lancet 1971;1: 1143-1145.

Bang HO, Dyerberg J, Hjorne N. The composition of food consumed by Greenland Eskimos. Acta Med Scand 1976;200: 69-73.

Bang HO, Dyerberg J, Sinclair HM. The composition of the Eskimo food in north western Greenland. Am J Clin Nutr 1980; 33:2657-2661.

Bates C, van Dam C, Horrobin DF, Morse N, Huang Y-S, Manku MS. Plasma essential fatty acids in pure and mixed race American Indians on and off a diet exceptionally rich in salmon. Porstaglandins Leukotrienes Med 1985;17:77-84.

Consensus Conference statement on lowering blood cholesterol to prevent heart disease. JAMA 1985;253:2080-2086.

Curb JD, Reed DM. Fish consumption and mortality from coronary heart disease. N Engl J Med 1985;313:821.

Dyerberg J, Bang HO. Haemostatic function and platelet polyunsaturated fatty acids in Eskimos. Lancet 1979;2:433-435.

Eskimo diets and diseases (Editorial). Lancet 1983;1:1139-1141.

Hebert PR, Fiebach NH, Eberlein KA, Taylor JO, Hennekens CH. The community-based randomized trials of pharmacological treatment of mild-to-moderate hypertension. Am J Epidemiol 1988;127:581-590.

Hennekens CH, Buring JE. Smoking and coronary disease in women. JAMA 1985;253:3003-3004.

Hennekens CH, Buring JE. Epidemiology in medicine. Boston: Little, Brown, 1987.

Hirai A, Hamazaki, T, Terano T et al. Eicosapentaenoic acid and platelet function in Japanese. Lancet 1980;2:1132-1133.

Illingworth 1987. Proceedings of conference.

Kagawa Y, Nishizawa M, Suzuki M et al. Eicosapolyenoic acids of serum lipids of Japanese Islanders with low incidence of cardiovascular diseases. J Nutr Sci Vitaminol 1982;28:441-453.

Kromann N, Green A. Epidemiological studies in the Upernavik District, Greenland. Incidence of some chronic diseases 1950-1974. Acta Med Scand 1980;208:401-406.

Kromhout D, Bosschieter EB, Coulander CdeL. The inverse relation between fish consumption and 20-year mortality from coronary heart disease. N Engl J Med 1985;312:1205-1209.

Shekelle RB, Paul O, Shyrock AM, Stamler J. Fish consumption and mortality from coronary heart disease. N Engl J Med 1985;313:820.

Stansby ME. Nutritional properties of fish oils. World Rev Nutr Diet 1969;11:46-105.

US DHHS. The health consequences of smoking: cardiovascular disease. Rockville, MD: Office on Smoking and Health, 1983.

US DHHS. Prevention '84/'85. Washington, DC: Public Health Service Office, 1985.

Vollset SE, Heuch I, Bjelke E. Fish consumption and mortality from coronary heart disease. N Engl J Med 1985;313:820-821.

Wallace RB, Anderson RA. Blood lipids, lipid-related measures, and the risk of atherosclerotic cardiovascular disease. Epidemiol Rev 1987;9;95-119.

4
The Effects of Fish Oil on Connective Tissue Metabolism and Connective Tissue Disease

Roy Soberman
Harvard Medical School and Brigham and Women's Hospital
Boston, Massachusetts

INTRODUCTION

Rhematoid arthritis is a chronic inflammatory disease in joints, currently estimated to affect 2-5% of adult Americans over the age of 55 (Hochberg, 1981). The pathological changes resulting in the eventual destruction of the rheumatoid joint are considered to be mediated by inflammatory cells such as polymorphonuclear leukocytes (PMN) (McCarty, 1989) and monocytes (Snyderman, 1985), which are particularly prominent in the synovial fluid, and by the pannus (new tissue growth in the joint space), respectively, which contains mononuclear cells. Damage to the rheumatoid joint, in part, can be attributed to the generation of highly reactive reduced oxygen species and the release of lysosomal proteases, with eventual destruction of articular cartilage (Badway and Karnovsky, 1980; McCord, 1974; Barrett, 1981). Of the substances known to be chemotactic for PMN and monocytes, $5S,12R$-

-dihydroxy-6,14-*cis*-8,10-*trans*-11,14-*cis*-eicosatetraenoic acid
(leukotriene B_4, LTB_4) is perhaps the most potent yet described
to be active in situ although, based on in vitro studies (Goetzl
and Pickett, 1980; Palmer et al., 1980), the complement frag-
ment C5a may be comparable. LTB_4 has been shown to be
formed from endogenous membrane-derived arachidonic acid
(AA) following stimulation of PMN or monocytes with the calcium ionophore A23187 (Borgeat and Samuelsson, 1979), or with
unopsonized zymosan (Williams et al., 1984), or from beta-glucan
particles (Czop and Austen, 1985), which act via a transmembrane
stimulation mechanism. The compounds LTB_4 and 5-hydroxy-
6,8,11,14-eicosatetraenoic acid (5-HETE), a stable reduction product of 5-hydroperoxy-6,8,11,14-eicosatetraenoic acid (5-HPETE),
have been shown to be selectively increased in the joints of patients
with rheumatoid arthritis (Klickstein et al., 1980).

AA released from the membranes of PMN is acted on by the
enzyme 5-lipoxygenase (Rouzer and Samuelsson, 1985; Goetz
et al., 1985; Soberman et al., 1985) to form 5-HPETE, which is
converted by the same enzyme to 5,6-oxido-7,9-*trans*-11,14-*cis*-
eicosatetraenoic acid (leukotriene A_4, LTA_4) (Shimizu et al.,
1984; Rouzer et al., 1986). In PMN, LTA_4 undergoes hydrolysis
by a specific cytosolic epoxide hydrolase to form LTB_4 (Radmark et al., 1984), which is not only chemotactic but also stimu-
lates aggregation, lysosomal enzyme release, and O_2^- generation in
PMN (Showell et al., 1982). LTB_4 mediates its actions via specific high- and low-affinity receptors that are present on the surface
of PMN (Goldman and Goetzl, 1984; Lin et al., 1984). LTB_4 is
deactivated by chemotaxis by successive omega-oxidations of its
C_{20} carbon, resulting first in the formation of 20-OH LTB_4 and
then 20-COOH LTB_4 (Hansson et al., 1981; Jubiz, et al. 1982;
Powell, 1984; Shak and Goldstein, 1984); the initial step is carried
out by a novel cytochrome P450, LTB_4 20-hydroxylase, present
in the microsomes of PMN (Shak, 1985; Soberman et al., 1985).
Alternatively, in monocytes (Williams et al., 1984) and eosinophils
(Weller et al., 1983; Owen et al., 1986) LTB_4 can be conjugated
with reduced glutathione by the enzyme leukotriene C_4 (LTC_4)
synthetase (Yochimoto et al., 1985) to form 5*S*-hydroxy-6*R*-*S*-

glutathionyl-7,9-*trans*-11,14-*cis*-eicosatetraenoic acid (LTC$_4$).
LTC$_4$ can be converted by the action of gamma-glutamyl trans-
peptidase to 5*S*-hydroxy-6*R*-*S*-cysteinylglycyl-9-*trans*-11,14-*cis*-
eicosatetraenoic acid (leukotriene D$_4$, LTD$_4$) (Orning, 1982),
which is subsequently converted to 5*S*-hydroxy-6*R*-*S*-cysteinyl-
glycyl-9-*trans*-11-, 14-*cis*-eicosatetraenoic acid (leukotriene E$_4$,
LTE$_4$) by a variety of dipeptidases, including one present in PMN
(Lewis et al., 1980; Lee et al., 1983). All three products, LTC$_4$,
LTD$_4$, and LTE$_4$, promote endothelial cell contraction and trans-
udation of fluid (Drazen et al., 1980; Dahlen et al., 1981), thus
producing edema and facilitating chemotaxis of peripheral blood
phagocytes into an area of inflammation. LTC$_4$ and LTD$_4$ also
constrict arterioles (Dahlen et al., 1981) and perhaps larger portions of the arterial beds (Badr et al., 1984; Pfeffer et al., 1983),
possibly contributing to a compromise in tissue viability. It is
possible that interruption of AA conversion to the leukotrienes
could serve to ameliorate the inflammatory processes in the rheumatoid joint.

CURRENT THERAPIES

Current therapies aimed at the treatment of rheumatoid arthritis
can be divided into those of symptomatic benefit, such as nonsteroidal antiinflammatory agents; those that are disease-remitting,
such as gold salts, penicillamine, and hydroxychloroquine; and
those considered to be disease-inhibiting, such as certain cytotoxic
interventions including azathioprine and methotrexate (Lightfoot,
1985; Weinblatt et al., 1985). Salicylates and the other nonsteroidal antiinflammatory agents produce side effects, including gastric distress and related symptoms such as peptic ulcer disease, salt
and water retention, and interstitial nephritis. The use of disease-
remitting agents such as gold and penicillamine is associated with
skin reactions, renal toxicity, and marrow suppression. The cytotoxic agents cause bone marrow suppression and immunosuppres-
sion, and in the case of methotrexate, hypersensitivity, pneumo-
nitis, and liver abnormalities (Lightfoot, 1985; Weinblatt et al.,
1985; Anderson et al., 1974; Martinez-Maldonado et al., 1983;
Rosa and Brown, 1983; Richter, 1980). Thus, the development

of less toxic agents which can eliminate or reduce the use of these therapies is highly desirable.

Fatty acids present in the triglycerides of cold-water fish in relatively large amounts include the omega-3 fatty acids—5,8,11, 14,17, all cis-eicosapentaenoic acid (EPA) and 4,7,10,13,16,19, all cis-docosahexaenoic acid (DHA). That these fatty acids might modulate production of AA-derived mediators was suggested by the demonstration that EPA and DHA are poor substrates for cyclooxygenase and are competitive inhibitors of AA utilization (Culp et al., 1979; Needleman et al., 1979; Gryglewski et al., 1979; Corey et al., 1980). In addition, thromboxane A_3, a product of EPA metabolism by the cyclooxygenase pathway, has a significantly attenuated platelet-aggregating ability (Needleman et al., 1979; Gryglewski et al., 1979). The low incidence of cardiovascular disease and possibly rheumatoid arthritis seen in Greenland Eskimos, who have a diet rich in omega-3 fatty acids (Sinclair, 1980; Stansby, 1969) compared with appropriate control populations, led to studies in further populations of the effects of dietary ingestion of fish oil fatty acids on the incidence of cardiovascular disease, with attention to alteration of the amounts and functional properties of AA-derived metabolites. Putative benefits were related to the attenuation of platelet aggregation through impaired generation of thromboxane A_2 (Needleman et al., 1979; Gryglewski et al., 1979), with the production instead of thromboxane A_3; however, the putative beneficial process is most likely substantially more complex.

EPA AS A SUBSTRATE FOR 5-LIPOXYGENASE

Murphy et al. (1981) observed that P815 mastocytoma cells in tissue culture convert EPA into 5-lipoxygenase products of the omega-3 class. Since then it has been observed that EPA is a preferred substrate for 5-lipoxygenase. The initial reaction product is 5-hydroperoxy-6,8,11,14,17-eicosapentaenoic acid (5-HPEPE) (Soberman et al., 1985a,b), which is then converted by way of the 5,6-oxido-7,9-trans-11,14,17-cis-eicosapentaenoic acid (LTA_5) intermediate to either 5S-hydroxy-6R-S-glutathionyl-7,9-trans-

11,14,17-*cis*-eicosapentaenoic acid (LTC_5) (Hammarstrom, 1980) or 5S,12R-dihydroxy-6,14,17-*cis* 8,10-*trans*-eicosapentaenoic acid (LTB_5) (Lee et al., 1984a,b; Prescott, 1984), depending on the specific cell type. LTB_5, which is produced in vitro by PMN stimulated with the calcium ionophore A23187 in the presence of exogenous EPA (Lee et al., 1984a,b; Lee et al., 1985), or from endogenous membrane EPA ultimately derived from diet (Kremer et al., 1985), is structurally similar to LTB_4 but is markedly attenuated in its ability to induce chemotaxis (Lee et al., 1984a,b). The 22-carbon fatty acid with six double bonds DHA (Soberman et al., 1985a,b; Corey et al., 1983; Lee et al., 1984a,b) is a poor substrate for 5-lipoxygenase, being converted to its products (7-OH- and 4-OH-DHA) at rates less than 5% that of AA or EPA. Although preventive and therapeutic approaches are not synonymous, the total data, taken together, suggest that dietary enrichment with omega-3 fatty acids could be a potentially useful, relatively nontoxic, therapeutic modality in inhibiting the generation of active proinflammatory metabolies of AA produced from both the cyclooxygenase and 5-lipoxygenase pathways and substituting in some instances attenuated pentaene analogs such as LTB_5 and thromboxane A_3. These considerations in the development of nontoxic therapy described above led to further studies of EPA metabolism.

In preliminary studies, needed to define the chromatographic behavior of the pentaene leukotrienes, to standardize their radio-immunoassay, and to resolve pentaene from tetraene products (Lee et al., 1984a,b), it was observed that neutrophils stimulated with ionophore A23187 in the presence of EPA had decreased production of LTB_4 from endogenous AA and LTB_5 from exogenous EPA as compared with control cells stimulated in the presence of exogenous AA. The inhibition of total LTB (LTB_4 and LTB_5) formation appeared to be preferentially at the site of the epoxide hydrolase (Lee et al., 1984a,b). Release of [^{3}H]AA from prelabeled cells was not reduced and there was no decrement in the production of 5-HETE and 5-HEPE intermediates, the markers for the epoxide intermediates sequentially involved in generation of the end products of LTB_4 and LTB_5 (Lee et al., 1984a,b). These

observations are consistent with the findings of inactivation of
LTA_4 hydrolase during its interaction with substrate (Kremer
et al., 1985) and with the observation that LTA_5 reacts with
LTA_4 hydrolase at a rate of about 50% that of LTA_4 (Kremer
et al., 1987).

In contrast, in early studies with normal volunteers receiving
6 weeks of dietary supplementation with 18 g daily of MaxEPA
capsules, a commercially available fish oil concentrate, isolated
neutrophils showed inhibition of $[^3H]AA$ release, and the generation of markers for both the 5-lipoxygenase steps and that of the
epxoide hydrolase (Lee et al., 1985) was suppressed. Thus, in
working with human PMN activated with a calcium ionophore, the
apparent mechanisms of impaired elaboration of LTB_4 were different when the alternative fatty acids were added and were
largely exogenous, and when they are ingested and endogenous.
Whether there is the same pattern of alteration of AA metabolism
as seen with ionophore when the agonist is a transmembrane stimulus remains to be elucidated.

PMN obtained from volunteers ingesting marine unsaturated
fatty acids on a regular basis as a part of their diet showed decreased chemotaxis in response to LTB_4 (58) (Lee et al., 1985)
under conditions where membrane fluidity was unchanged.
Whether a specific functional deficiency in response to such factors occurs in receptor binding or in the metabolic steps initiated
at the receptor level is not known. Possibilities for the latter include coupling to or activation of phosphatidyl-inositol-4,5-*bis*-
phosphate-specific phosphodiesterase, as for N-formyl-L-meth-
ionyl-L-leucyl-L-phenylalanine (FMLP), or the mobilization of
intracellular calcium, seen in response to LTB_4.

In a recent study of the effects of ingesting 18 g/day of
MaxEPA on multiple metabolic parameters in nine normal,
healthy volunteers, Endress et al. (1989) showed that fish oil
ingestion produced a marked fall in the production in vitro by
the subjects' mononuclear cells of two inflammatory cytokines,
interleukin-1 and tumor necrosis factor (TNF). Furthermore,
10 weeks after the end of the 6-week period of dietary fish oil
supplementation, the inhibitionof inflammatory cytokine produc-

tion was even greater than it was at the 6-week time point. The authors conclude that the antiinflammatory effects of fish oil supplementation may be mediated in part by an inhibition of the production of the inflammatory cytokines interleukin-1 and TNF.

The effects of dietary omega-3 fatty acids on the clinical course of rheumatoid arthritis and on the biochemical properties of peripheral blood leukocytes taken from rheumatoid patients has been examined by two groups. Sperling and co-workers (1987) fed 12 patients with active rheumatoid arthritis 20 g daily of MaxEPA for 6 weeks with the incorporation of EPA into cellular lipids of PMN and monocytes documented by gas chromatography. At 6 weeks, a parameter of clinical improvement, the joint-pain index, decreased significantly, as compared with the pre-diet period. However, no significant change in 5-lipoxygenase product generation was observed, though platelet-activating factor generation by monocytes stimulated with the calcium ionophore A23187 decreased significantly at week 6. Though PMN chemotaxis to both LTB_4 and FMLP was suppressed at the beginning of the study, by week 6, PMN chemotaxis returned to levels seen in healthy volunteers, even though the patients were still taking the fish oil capsules. The reason for this is not clear. Kremer and co-workers have concluded three trials of the effects of dietary marine fatty acids in rheumatoid arthritis (Kremer et al., 1985, 1987, 1988). These trials were placebo-controlled using olive oil as the placebo. The authors demonstrated a statistically significant improvement in several clinical parameters and a decrease in PMN generation of LTB_4 by the patient group.

SUMMARY

In summary, an increasing body of evidence derived from in vitro studies suggests that fish oil supplementation and/or fish oil fatty acids inhibit a number of the biochemical mediators of the inflammatory process, particularly parameters known to be pertinent to rheumatoid arthritis. These studies include not only animal studies, but also studies of white cells from human subjects whose diet has been supplemented with fish oil concentrate. Unfortunately, the large body of biochemical data has not yet been accompanied by an equal number of randomized trials of the clinical effects of fish oil on arthritis. However, the few studies that have been published suggest that dietary supplementation with large amounts of fish oil may decrease joint pain, increase mobility, and generally improve both the subjective and objective parameters of rheumatoid joint disease. To date, the data are still fragmentary and grossly inadequate to support any general recommendation that patients with rheumatoid or other forms of arthritis be treated with fish oil rather than more established therapy. Therefore, it is crucial to obtain the clinical evidence that will allow us to assess the appropriate role of fish oil and fish oil fatty acids in the treatment of the rheumatoid diseases.

ACKNOWLEDGMENT

The work was funded by Grants AR-38638 and AI-22563 from the National Institutes of Health and a Grant-in-Aid from the American Heart Association, with funds contributed in part by the Massachusetts chapter.

REFERENCES

Anderson RJ, Berl T, McDonald K, Schrer RW. J Clin Invest 1974;53:69.

Badr KF, Baylis C, Pfeffer JM et al. Circ Res 1984;54:492.

Badway JA, Karnovsky ML. Annu Rev Biochem 1980;49:695.

Barrett AJ. Semin Arthritis Rheum 1981;11:52.

Borgeat P, Samuelsson B. Proc Natl Acad Sci USA 1979;76:2148.

Corey EJ, Shih C, Cashman JR. Proc Natl Acad Sci USA 1983; 80:3581-3584.

Culp BR, Titus BG, Lands WEM. Prostaglandins Med 1979;3:269.

Czop JK, Austen KF. J Immunol 1985;82:6040.

Dahlen SE, Hedqvist PM, Hammerstrom S, Samuelsson B. Proc Natl Acad Sci USA 1981;78:3887.

Drazen JM, Austen KF, Lewis RA et al. Proc Natl Acad Sci USA 1980;77:4354.

Endress S, Ghorbani R, Kelley VE, et al. N Engl J Med 1989; 320;265-271.

Goetze A, Fayer L, Bouska J, Dommerer D, Carter GW. Prostaglandins 1985;29:689.

Goetzl EJ, Pickett W. J Immunol 1980;125:1789.

Goldman DW, Goetzl EJ. J Exp Med 1984;159:1027.

Gryglewski RJ, Salmon JA, Ubatruba FB. Weatherly BC, Moncada S, Vane JR. Prostaglandins 1979;18:453.

Hammarstrom S. J Biol Chem 1980;255:7093.

Hansson G, Lindgren J-A, Dahlen S-E, Hedqvist P, Samuelsson B. FEBS Lett 1981;130:107.

Hochberg MC. Epidemiol Rev 1981;3:27.

Jubiz W, Radmark O, Malmstem C, et al. J Biol Chem 1982;257: 6106.

Klickstein LB, Shapleigh C, Goetzl EJ. J Clin Invest 1980;66: 1166.

Kremer JM, Bigauoette J, Michalek AV, et al. Lancet 1985;1:184-187.

Kremer JM, Jubiz W, Michalek A, et al. Ann Intern Med 1987; 106:497-503.

Kremer JM, Lawrence D, Jubiz W, Digiacomo R, Rynes R, Bartholomew L. Arthritis Rheum 1988;31:530.

Lee CW, Lewis RA, Carey EJ, Austen KF. Immunology 1983; 48:27.

Lee TH, Mencia-Huerta J-M, Shih C, Corey EJ, Lewis RA, Austen KF. J Biol Chem 1984a;259:2383.

Lee TH, Mencia-Huerta J-M, Shih C, Corey EJ, Lewis RA, Austen KF. J Clin Invest 1984b;74:1922.

Lee TH, Hoover RL, Williams JD, et al. N Engl J Med 1985;312: 1217.

Lewis RA, Drazen JM, Austen KF, Clark DA, Corey EJ. Biochem Biophys Res Commun 1980;96:271.

Lightfoot RW Jr. In: McCarty DJ, et al. eds. Arthritis. Philadelphia, Lea & Febiger, 1985: 668.

Lin AH, Ruppel PL, Gorman RR. Prostaglandins 1984;28:837.

Martinez-Maldonado, Benabe JE, Lopez-Novoa. In Lazarus JM, Brenner BM, eds. Acute renal failure. Philadelphia: Saunders, 1983: 434.

McCarty DJ. In: McCarty DJ, et al, eds. Arthritis. Philadelphia: Lea & Febiger, 1989: 74.

McCord JM. Science 1974;185:529.

Murphy RC, Pickett WC, Culp BR, Land WEM. Prostaglandins 1981;22:613.

Needleman P, Raz A, Mnkes MS, Ferrendelli JA, Sprecher H. Proc Natl Acad Sci USA 1979;76:944.

Orning L, Hammarstrom S. Biochem Biophys Res Commun 1982; 106:1304.

Owen WF, Silberstein DS, Soberman RJ, et al. In: Proceedings of the Sixth International Congress of Immunology, 1986.

Palmer RJM, Stephney RJ, Higgs GA, Eakins KE. Prostaglandins 1980;20:411.

Pfeffer MA, Pfeffer JM, Lewis RA, Braunwald E, Corey EJ, Austen KF. Am J Physiol 1983;224:628H.

Powell WS. J Biol Chem 1984;259:3082.

Prescott SM. J Biol Chem 1984;259:7615.

Radmark O, Shimizu T, Jornvall H, Samuelsson B. J Biol Chem 1984;254:12339.

Richter JA, et al. J Rheumatol 1980;7:153.

Rosa RM, Brown RS. In: Lazarus JM, Brenner BM, eds. Acute renal failure. Philadelphia: Saunders, 1983: 434.

Rouzer CA, Samuelsson B. Proc Natl Acad Sci USA 1985;82: 6040.

Rouzer CA, Matsumoto T, Samuelsson B. Proc Natl Acad Sci USA 1986;83:857.

Samuelsson B. J Biol Chem 1982;257:6106.

Shak S, Goldstein IM. J Biol Chem 1984;259:10181.

Shak S, Goldstein IM. J Clin Invest 1985;76:1218.

Shimizu T, Radmark O, Samuelsson B. Proc Natl Acad Sci USA 1984;81:689.

Showell HG, Naccache PH, Borgeat P, et al. J Immunol 1982;128: 811.

Sinclair HM. In Fumagalli R, Kritchevsky D, Paoletti R, eds. Drugs affecting lipid metabolism. Amsterdam: Elsevier North Holland Biomedical Press, 1980: 363.

Snyderman R. In: McCarty DJ, et al, eds. Arthritis. Philadelphia: Lea & Febiger, 1985: 287.

Soberman RJ, Harper TW, Betteridge D, Lewis RA, Austen KF. J Biol Chem 1985a;260:4508.

Soberman RJ, Harper TW, Murphy RC, Austen KF. Proc Natl Acad Sci USA 1985b;82:2292.

Sperling RI, Weinblatt M, Robin J-L, et al. Arthritis Rheum 1987; 30:988-997.

Stansby NE. World Rev Nutr Dietet 1969;11:46.

Weinblatt ME, Coblyn JS, Fox DA, et al. N Engl J Med 1985;312: 818.

Weller PF, Lee CW, Foster DW, Corey EJ, Lewis RA, Austen KF. Proc Natl Acad Sci USA 1983;80:7626.

Williams JD, Czop JK, Austen KF. J Immunol 1984;132:2024.

Yoshimoto T, Soberman RJ, Lewis RA, Austen KF. Proc Natl Acad Sci USA 1985;82:2292.

5
Experimental and Epidemiological Evidence on Marine Lipids and Carcinogenesis

Kenneth K. Carroll
University of Western Ontario
London, Ontario, Canada

INTRODUCTION

Experimental evidence that dietary fat can influence carcinogenesis has been accumulating for more than 50 years. The early studies showed that skin cancer and mammary cancer developed more readily in rodents fed high-fat diets compared to those fed low-fat diets (Watson and Mellanby, 1930; Baumann et al., 1939; Tannenbaum, 1942). In these early studies, various types of fat were used, but there was little attempt to compare the effects of different types of fat (Carroll and Khor, 1975; Carroll, 1986a).

Interest in this area of research revived during the 1970s as a result of further studies on experimental tumor models coupled with epidemiological evidence of positive correlations between dietary fat and cancer incidence and mortality (Armstrong and Doll, 1975; Carroll and Khor, 1975). The new experimental data showed that polyunsaturated vegetable oils increased the yields of

mammary tumors (Carroll and Khor, 1971), pancreatic tumors
(Roebuck et al., 1981), and possibly intestinal tumors (Reddy and
Maeura, 1984) more effectively than saturated fats. Studies on
mammary tumors also indicated that polyunsaturated fats were
more effective because of their higher content of linoleic acid,
which seems to be required for enhancement of tumor yields
(Hopkins et al., 1981; Ip, 1987).

Studies with prostaglandin synthesis inhibitors (Hillyard
and Abraham, 1979; Carter et al., 1983) suggested that effects
of polyunsaturated vegetable oils on mammary tumorigenesis
were mediated by eicosanoids of the 2-series derived from linoleic
acid. Dietary fish oils might therefore be expected to have different effects since their polyunsaturated fatty acids belong mainly
to the n-3 family and give rise to eicosanoids of the 3-series,
which can differ in physiological properties from those of the 2-
series. Fatty acids of the n-3 family can also compete with linoleic acid and other fatty acids of the n-6 family for enzymes involved in the steps leading to eicosanoids and may thus inhibit
formation of the 2-series of eicosanoids (Oliw et al., 1983).
These considerations led us to investigate the effects of dietary
fish oil on mammary tumorigenesis in rats (Carroll and Braden,
1985).

Another stimulus for such investigations came from studies
on Greenland Eskimos which indicated that they suffer less from
cardiovascular disease and other chronic diseases, including cancer,
than might be expected on the basis of the high-fat diet they consume (Dyerberg, 1986; Carroll, 1986b). Marine animals, including
seals, whales, and fish, make up a large proportion of this diet
(Bang et al., 1976), and much of the interest has centered on the
fat component of the diet, which contains substantial amounts of
n-3 fatty acids (Dyerberg, 1986). Fish are also an important
component of the Japanese diet, and evidence of low mortality
from breast cancer in the Eskimo and Japanese populations led
Karmali et al. (1984) to study the effects of dietary fish oil on
mammary cancer in rats.

This chapter is concerned with recent experimental and
epidemiological evidence on marine lipids and carcinogenesis.

EXPERIMENTAL STUDIES

Mammary Cancer

Transplanted Tumors

For their studies, Karmali et al. (1984) used female F344 rats implanted with 3-mm^3 pieces of R323OAC mammary adenocarcinoma. The rats were fed chow diet and given oral supplements of 100, 200, or 400 μl/rat/day of a fish oil concentrate (MaxEPA) containing 17 mg of eicosapentaenoic acid (EPA) and 16 mg of docosahexaenoic acid (DHA) per 100 μl. The smallest dose reduced tumor weight and volume by about one-third after 4 weeks of treatment, and similar results were obtained with the higher doses. EPA and DHA accumulated in the choline phospholipids of the tumors, and the tumor content and in vitro synthesis of prostaglandins were reduced by the treatment.

The results of subsequent experiments in which MaxEPA and corn oil were added to semipurified diets alone or in combination gave less clear-cut results (Karmali, 1987a,b). Although there was a marginal reduction in tumor size with a 1:1 mixture of MaxEPA and corn oil fed at the 23.5% level, the group fed fish oil alone had larger tumors than those fed corn oil alone at this level.

Gabor and Abraham (1986) compared the effects of diets containing 10% hydrogenated cottonseed oil (HCTO), corn oil, or menhaden oil on growth of mammary adenocarcinoma IX transplanted into BALB/c mice. The fish oil used for these experiments contained approximately 1% linoleic acid, 16% EPA, and 11% DHA. The tumors grew more slowly in mice fed the HCTO or menhaden oil compared to those fed corn oil. Menhaden oil was more effective than HCTO in counteracting the growth-promoting effects of corn oil, but the effect only became apparent at a ratio of 9 parts of menhaden oil to 1 part of corn oil. These results were interpreted as supporting the idea that prostaglandins are involved in the regulation of mammary tumor mass. Analysis of the fatty acid composition of liver and tumor lipids from animals on these diets showed changes in line with the fatty acid composition of the dietary fat. The rate at which cells were lost from tumors of mice fed the corn oil diet was less than half of that observed for tumors of mice fed HCTO or menhaden oil. The lower weight of tumors on the latter diets may therefore be due to an increased rate of cell loss rather than a decreased rate of cell production.

Adams and Karmali (1987) provided some evidence that dietary fish oil has an inhibitory effect on growth of metastatic foci from mammary tumors (see also Karmali, 1987b). They studied the effects of diets containing 23.5% corn oil; 8% corn oil and 15.5% fish oil; 3% corn oil and 20.5% fish oil; and 5% corn oil on 13762 MAT:B mammary tumor in an artificial metastasis system. Studies were also done on 13762 NF mammary tumor in a spontaneous metastasis model. Preliminary results with the artificial metastasis system showed that tumor volume and frequency were decreased by the diets containing fish oil. Tumor volumes for the two fish oil diets were intermediate between those for the diets containing 23.5% and 5% corn oil.

Reitz et al. (1987) implanted approximately 1 mm^3 of MX-1 human mammary carcinoma cells into athymic nude mice by trochar and found that the tumor growth rate was statistically slower in mice fed a 10% cod liver oil diet compared to those fed a 10% corn oil diet. The diets were fed for 21 days before and 24-31 days after implantation of the tumor cells.

Chemically Induced Tumors

Effects of dietary menhaden oil on chemically induced mammary tumorigenesis have also been compared with those of corn oil. Jurkowski and Cave (1985) investigated effects on mammary tumors induced by N-methyl-N-nitrosourea (NMU) in female BUF rats, whereas experiments in our laboratory were done on mammary tumors induced by 7,12-dimethylbenz(a)anthracene (DMBA) in female Sprague-Dawley rats (Braden and Carroll, 1986). In both cases, menhaden oil fed at higher levels (10 or 20% by weight) suppressed tumorigenesis, whereas at low levels (0.5 or 3%) the rats fed menhaden oil were more prone to develop tumors than those fed the same level of corn oil. In an earlier study in our laboratory in which a diet containing 3% menhaden oil and 17% coconut oil was fed to rats given DMBA, a marked stimulation of tumorigenesis was observed relative to that in rats fed a diet containing 20% coconut oil (Hopkins et al., 1981).

Jurkowski and Cave (1985) analyzed the microsomal fatty acid composition of tumors and of livers from rats fed the different diets and observed changes in the n-3 and n-6 fatty acids consistent with the levels of those fatty acids in the dietary fats. In a more recent study, Cave and Jurkowski (1987) compared the effects of diets containing 15% corn oil and 5% menhaden oil or 5% corn oil and 15% menhaden oil with those obtained by feeding either oil at the 20% level. The results showed that replacing 5% of the corn oil by menhaden oil had little effect on tumorigenesis while replacement of 15% of the corn oil gave results that were intermediate between those obtained with corn oil and menhaden oil alone. Fatty acid analysis of the tumor microsomal lipids again showed a positive correlation between the proportion of linoleic acid and the amount of corn oil in the diet and a positive correlation between the proportion of EPA and the amount of dietary menhaden oil. The groups fed large amounts of menhaden oil had more phosphatidylserine and phosphatidylethanolamine in the membranes and less phosphatidylcholine than those fed large amounts of corn oil.

Ip et al. (1986) compared the effects on DMBA-induced mammary tumorigenesis of diets containing 20% corn oil, 12% menhaden oil plus 8% corn oil, and 19% menhaden oil plus 1% corn oil. The lowest tumor incidence and yield were observed on the diet containing 12% menhaden oil and 8% corn oil. The authors interpreted this to mean that observed inhibitory effects of this fish oil on mammary tumorigenesis were not due to its low content of linoleic acid and consequent deficiency of n-6 essential fatty acid. They also reported that mammary tumors had a greater tendency to regress in animals fed the fish oil diets.

Colon Cancer

The effects of dietary menhaden oil on tumors of the large bowel induced by axoxymethane in male F344 rats were investigated by

Reddy and Maruyama (1986). The animals were fed a diet containing 5% corn oil until after administration of the carcinogen. They were then transferred to diets containing 4% menhaden oil plus 1% corn oil; 22.5% menhaden oil plus 1% corn oil; or 23.5% corn oil. One group was continued on the 5% corn oil diet. The animals were examined endoscopically at 20 and 30 weeks and were autopsied 34 weeks after the last injection of carcinogen.

The incidence and multiplicity of adenomas and adenocarcinomas in the large intestine were lower in the groups fed diets containing menhaden oil or the low level of corn oil than in those fed the high corn oil diet. The incidence of adenomas and adenocarcinomas localized in the duodenum, and of squamous cell carcinomas of the ear duct, was not significantly different among animals in the different dietary groups. Body weight was lower in the group fed the high level of menhaden oil but was similar in the other dietary groups. It is possible that the differing effects of menhaden oil and corn oil are related to differences in eicosanoid production since earlier studies had shown that indomethacin has an inhibitory effect on chemically induced large bowel carcinogenesis in rats (Pollard and Luckert, 1981; Narisawa et al., 1982).

Effects of dietary corn oil and menhaden oil on colon cancer induced in rats by 1,2-dimethylhydrazine (DMH) have been investigated by Nelson et al. (1987). For this purpose, two groups of 19 male Sprague-Dawley rats were fed chow diets to which were added corn oil or menhaden oil, respectively, so that fat provided 37% of ingested calories. After 1 week on diet, the rats were given six weekly injections of 20 mg/kg DMH subcutaneously. The animals were killed 4 months after the last injection and rats fed the menhaden oil diet were found to have significantly fewer tumors than those fed the corn oil diet. However, the incidence of colorectal tumors was not significantly different between the two groups. Plasma hydroperoxides were analyzed 4 weeks after the last DMH treatment but failed to show any significant differences among the dietary groups.

Broitman et al. (1987) recently compared the effects of dietary safflower oil and menhaden oil fed at levels of 5 and 20% on growth and pulmonary colonization of a transplantable colon carcinoma, CT-26, implanted into the intestine of mice. They reported that tumor growth was inhibited by menhaden oil at both levels of intake and that colonization of the lung was also inhibited by the 20% menhaden oil diet.

Pancreatic Cancer

O'Connor et al. (1985) studied the effects of fish oil and fish protein on preneoplastic atypical acinar cell nodules (AACN) of rat pancreas induced by L-azaserine. The three diets used contained 20% casein and 20% corn oil; 21.1% freeze-dried cod and 20% corn oil; and 21.1% cod and 20% menhaden oil, respectively. At 14 days of age rats were given 30 mg/kg body weight of L-azaserine and 1 week later they were weaned to the respective diets. Four months later they were killed and the number of lesions was determined by histological examination of the pancreas.

Comparison of the results for the first two diets indicated that the fish protein had no significant effect on pancreatic lesions, whereas the third diet, containing menhaden oil, markedly reduced the number and size of lesions. No carcinomas were observed in the fish oil group compared to six in the group fed fish protein and corn oil and three in the group fed casein and corn oil. There was a total of 16 animals in each dietary group.

In a subsequent study, O'Connor et al. (1987) investigated the effect of diets containing mixtures of corn oil and menhaden oil in different proportions (20/0, 19/1, 17/3, 15/5, 10/10, 5/15, 3/17, 1/19, and 0/20). In each case, fat made up 20% of the diet and the dietary protein was provided by freeze-dried cod. The experimental protocol was the same as that used in the earlier experiment. The results showed that the % volume of pancreas occupied by AACN began to decrease when the menhaden oil was increased from 5 to 10% and showed the greatest decrease between 10 and 15% menhaden oil. The ratios of omega-3 to omega-6 fatty acids in these two diets were 0.41 and 1.2, respectively. Diets containing 15% or more of menhaden oil all gave similar results.

Prostatic Cancer

Effects of dietary fish oil on prostatic cancer have been studied to
a limited extent. Karmali et al. (1986) monitored the growth of
1×10^6 DU-145 human prostatic carcinoma cells inoculated subcutaneously into 4-6-week-old male, Swiss nu/nu mice fed diets
containing 23.5% corn oil or 20.5% MaxEPA plus 3% corn oil.
They found that tumor growth was significantly less in mice on
the fish oil diet at the end of the experiment.

EPIDEMIOLOGICAL EVIDENCE

As mentioned in the Introduction, epidemiological evidence of
low cancer mortality in populations such as Eskimos and Japanese
provided a stimulus to experimental studies on effects of dietary
fish oils on carcinogenesis. Karmali et al. (1984) cited reports by
Doll et al. (1966), Berg (1975), and Nielsen and Hansen (1980)
that Eskimos and Japanese have a low mortality from breast cancer. (For more recent data on cancer incidence in Japan see
Waterhouse et al., 1982.) They also noted that risk of breast cancer in Greenland is not correlated with total fat intake since fat
consumption by Greenland Eskimos is comparable to that in Denmark, where breast cancer is more prevalent. There is also evidence that the incidence of breast cancer in Greenland and Iceland rose following a period when the dietary habits became
Westernized (Bjarnason et al., 1974; Nielsen and Hansen, 1980)
and that breast and colon cancer rates have risen in Japan in recent
years as fat consumption has increased (Hirayama, 1979). In
addition, Reddy and Maruyama (1986) cited evidence that Alaskan Eskimos have lower cancer rates than American whites or
other Western populations, although this only applies to cancer
at certain sites (Blot et al., 1975; Lanier et al., 1980).

In contrast to the above findings, Kromann and Green (1980)
reported that overall cancer incidence in a study population of
approximtely 1800 Eskimos during the 25 years from 1950 to
1974 was only 10-15% lower than expected from data for Denmark. Breast cancer and gastrointestinal cancer rates were about

the same as for the Danish population. In the same Eskimo population, incidence of myocardial infarction and bronchial asthma was less than 10% of that in Denmark. Diabetes was also relatively uncommon, and no cases of thyrotoxicosis or multiple sclerosis were observed. Although cancer rates increased during the latter half of the period and the population was probably become more Westernized, these data suggest that the lifestyle of the population had much less effect on cancer than on other chronic diseases. Even in cases where cancer incidence has been observed to be lower than expected, the difference may not necessarily be due to diet. For example, Hildes and Schaefer (1984) suggested that the lower incidence of breast cancer in Canadian Inuit was probably due to their practice of suckling infants for relatively long periods of time.

In a prospective study on a large group of married female registered nurses, Stampfer et al. (1987) found no significant differences in risk of breast cancer between those who ate fish once per month or less and those who ate up to two or more portions per week.

SUMMARY AND CONCLUSIONS

From recent studies on cancer in experimental animals it is clear that diets containing high levels of fish oil do not promote development of tumors of the mammary gland, colon, and pancreas. Their effects on tumorigenesis are thus different from those of diets containing high levels of polyunsaturated vegetable oils. The polyunsaturated fatty acids of fish oils belong mainly to the n-3 family, whereas linoleic acid, an n-6 fatty acid, is the major polyunsaturated fatty acid of vegetable oils. Linoleic acid appears to be required for promotion of tumorigenesis by dietary vegetable oils and the effect can be abolished by prostaglandin synthesis inhibitors. It has therefore been suggested that eicosanoids derived from linoleic acid mediate tumor promotion and that the n-3 fatty acids in fish oils do not promote because they inhibit the formation of eicosanoids from linoleic acid (Karmali et al., 1984; Reddy, 1987).

Although this is an appealing hypothesis, recent studies of Carter et al. (1987) have shown that carprofen, a prostaglandin synthesis inhibitor, fails to prevent the enhancement of mammary tumor incidence and yield in rats fed a high corn oil diet. There is also some evidence that diets containing low levels of fish oil or polyunsaturated vegetable oil have similar effects on mammary tumorigenesis (Hopkins et al., 1981; Jurkowski and Cave, 1985; Braden and Carroll, 1986). The polyunsaturated fatty acids in fish oils are oxidized more readily than those in vegetable oils (Cho et al., 1987) and products of such oxidation are known to have toxic effects on cells (Flower, 1979; Bird et al., 1982) which could possibly account for the inhibitory effects of high levels of dietary fish oils on tumorigenesis (Braden and Carroll, 1986).

Epidemiological studies have provided evidence that cancer is less prevalent in Eskimos consuming high-fat diets derived mainly from marine animals than in other populations whose diet contains comparable levels of fat from land animals and plants. The Japanese also consume relatively large amounts of marine lipids and have a lower cancer incidence than many Western nations, but the total fat intake of the Japanese is also lower and this could affect cancer incidence. Furthermore, some of the epidemiological data on Eskimos suggest that the differences in their susceptibility to cancer relative to other populations are less than for cardiovascular disease, bronchial asthma, diabetes, and other chronic diseases (Kromann and Green, 1980).

As indicated above, dietary fish oils do not promote tumorigenesis in animals, as do polyunsaturated vegetable oils. However, when mixtures of fish oil and polyunsaturated vegetable oil are fed, the results indicate that the diets promote tumorigenesis until a relatively high ratio of fish oil to vegetable oil is reached (Cave and Jurkowski, 1987; O'Connor et al., 1987). Thus, the combined experimental and epidemiological evidence suggests that dietary fish oil is unlikely to have a marked effect on cancer incidence in humans at moderate levels of intake. However, further investigation is warranted. In particular, comparative studies on effects of fish oil and other types of fats and oils on cancer in experimental animals may help to shed light on the mechanisms by which dietary fat influences carcinogenesis.

REFERENCES

Adams LM, Karmali RA. Inhibition of artificial metastasis in rat mammary tumor 13762 by dietary fish oil. Fed Proc 1987; 46:437 (Abstr. 703).

Armstrong B, Doll R. Environmental factors and cancer incidence and mortality in different countries, with special reference to dietary practices. Int J Cancer 1975;15:617-631.

Bang HO, Dyerberg J, Hjørne N. The composition of food consumed by Greenland Eskimos. Acta Med Scand 1976;200: 69-73.

Baumann CA, Jacobi HP, Rusch HP. The effect of diet on experimental tumor production. Am J Hyg 1939;30A:1-6.

Berg JW. Can nutrition explain the pattern of international epidemiology of hormone-dependent cancers? Cancer Res 1975;35:3345-3350.

Bird RP, Draper HH, Valli VEO. Toxicological evaluation of malonaldehyde: a 12-month study of mice. J Toxicol Environ Health 1982;10:897-905.

Bjarnason O, Day N, Snaedal G, Tulinius H. The effect of year of birth on the breast cancer age-incidence curve in Iceland. Int J Cancer 1974;13:689-696.

Blot WJ, Lanier A, Fraumeni JF Jr, Bender TR. Cancer mortality among Alaskan natives, 1960-69. J Natl Cancer Inst 1975; 55:547-554.

Braden LA, Carroll KK. Dietary polyunsaturated fat in relation to mammary carcinogenesis in rats. Lipids 1986;21:285-288.

Broitman SA, Cannizzo F, Rogers A, Gottlieb LS. Comparison of dietary marine oil and safflower oil on growth and pulmonary colonization of CT-26 implanted into bowel of mice. Fed Proc 1987;46:437 (Abstr. 704).

Carroll KK. Diet and carcinogenesis: historical perspectives. In: Poirier LA, Newberne PM, Pariza MW, eds. Adv. Exp. Med. Biol. Vol. 206. Essential nutrients in carcinogenesis. New York: Plenum Press, 1986a: 45-53.

Carroll KK. Biological effects of fish oils in relation to chronic diseases. Lipids 1986b;21:731-732.

Carroll KK, Braden LM. Dietary fat and mammary carcinogenesis. Nutr Cancer 1985;6:254-259.

Carroll KK, Khor HT. Effects of level and type of dietary fat on incidence of mammary tumors induced in female Sprague-Dawley rats by 7,12-dimethylbenz(a)anthracene. Lipids 1971;6:415-420.

Carroll KK, Khor HT. Dietary fat in relation to tumorigenesis. Prog Biochem Pharmacol 1975;10:308-353.

Carter CA, Milholland RJ, Shea W, Ip MM. Effect of the prostaglandin synthetase inhibitor indomethacin on 7,12-dimethylbenz(a)anthracene-induced mammary tumorigenesis in rats fed different levels of fat. Cancer Res 1983;43:3559-3562.

Carter CA, Ip MM, Ip C. Response of mammary carcinogenesis to dietary linoleate and fat levels and its modulation by prostaglandin synthesis inhibitors. In: Lands WEM, ed. Proc. AOCS short course on polyunsaturated fatty acids and eicosinoids. Champaign, IL: American Oil Chemists' Society, 1987: 253-260.

Cave WT Jr, Jurkowski JJ. Comparative effects of omega-3 and omega-6 dietary lipids on rat mammary tumor development. In: Lands WEM, ed. Proc. AOCS short course on polyunsaturated fatty acids and eicosanoids. Champaign, IL: American Oil Chemists' Society, 1987: 261-266.

Cho S-Y, Miyashita K, Miyazawa T, Fujimoto K, Kaneda T. Autooxidation of ethyl eicosapentaenoate and docosahexaenoate. J Am Oil Chemists' Soc 1987;64:876-879.

Doll R, Payne P, Waterhouse J. Cancer incidence in five continents. Berlin: Springer-Verlag, 1966.

Dyerberg J. Linolenate-derived polyunsaturated fatty acids and prevention of atherosclerosis. Nutr Rev 1986;44:125-134.

Flower RJ. Biosynthesis of prostaglandins. In: Oxygen free radicals and tissue damage. Ciba Foundation Symposium 65. Amsterdam: Excerpta Medica, 1979: 123-142.

Gabor H, Abraham S. Effect of dietary menhaden oil on tumor cell loss and the accumulation of mass of a transplantable mammary adenocarcinoma in BALB/c mice. J Natl Cancer Inst 1986;76:1223-1229.

Hildes JA, Schaefer O. The changing picture of neoplastic disease in the western and central Canadian Arctic (1950-1980). Can Med Assoc J 1984;130:25-32.

Hillyard LA, Abraham S. Effect of dietary polyunsaturated fatty acids on growth of mammary adenocarcinomas in mice and rats. Cancer Res 1979;39:4430-4437.

Hirayama T. Diet and cancer. Nutr Cancer 1979;1(3):67-81.

Hopkins GJ, Kennedy TG, Carroll KK. Polyunsaturated fatty acids as promoters of mammary carcinogenesis induced in Sprague-Dawley rats by 7,12-dimethylbenz(a)anthracene. J Natl Cancer Inst 1981;66:517-522.

Ip C. Fat and essential fatty acid in mammary carcinogenesis. Am J Clin Nutr 1987;45(Suppl):218-224.

Ip C, Ip MM, Sylvester P. Relevance of trans fatty acids and fish oil in animal tumorigenesis studies. In: Prog Clin Biol Res Vol 222, Dietary fat and cancer, Ip C, Birt DF, Rogers AE, Mettlin C, eds. New York: Alan R Liss, 1986: 283-294.

Jurkowski JJ, Cave WT Jr. Dietary effects of menhaden oil on the growth and membrane lipid composition of rat mammary tumors. J Natl Cancer Inst 1985;74:1145-1150.

Karmali RA. Fatty acids: inhibition. Am J Clin Nutr 1987a;45 (Suppl):225-229.

Karmali RA. Omega-3 fatty acids and cancer: a review. In: Lands WEM, ed. Proc AOCS short course on polyunsaturated fatty acids and eicosanoids. Champaign, IL: American Oil Chemists' Society, 1987b: 222-232.

Karmali RA, Marsh J, Fuchs C. Effect of omega-3 fatty acids on growth of a rat mammary tumor. J Natl Cancer Inst 1984; 73:457-461.

Karmali RA, Reichel P, Cohen LA. Dietary effects of omega-3 fatty acids on the growth of the DU-145 prostatic tumor. Fed Proc 1986;45:236 (Abstr. 477).

Kromann N, Green A. Epidemiological studies in the Upernavik District, Greenland. Acta Med Scand 1980;208:401-406.

Lanier AP, Blot WJ, Bender TR, Fraumeni JP Jr. Cancer in Alaskan Indians, Eskimos, and Aleuts. J Natl Cancer Inst 1980; 65:1157-1159.

Narisawa T, Sato M, Sano M, Takahashi T. Inhibition of development of methylnitrosourea-induced rat colonic tumors by peroral administration of indomethacin. Gann 1982;73:377-381.

Nelson RL, Tanure JC, Andrianopoulos G, Souza G, Lands WEM. A comparison of dietary fish body oil and corn oil in experimental colorectal carcinogenesis. In: Lands WEM, ed. Proc. AOCS short course on polyunsaturated fatty acids and eicosanoids. Champaign, IL: American Oil Chemists' Society, 1987: 518-522.

Nielsen NH, Hansen JPH. Breast cancer in Greenland—selected epidemiological, clinical, and histological features. J Cancer Res Clin Oncol 1980;98:287-299.

O'Connor TP, Roebuck BD, Peterson F, Campbell TC. Effect of dietary intake of fish oil and fish protein on the development of L-azaserine-induced preneoplastic lesions in the rat pancreas. J Natl Cancer Inst 1985;75:959-962.

O'Connor TP, Roebuck BD, Campbell TC. Effect of varying dietary omega-3:omega-6 fatty acid ratio on L-azaserine induced preneoplastic development in rat pancreas. In: Lands WEM, ed. Proc. AOCS short course on polyunsaturated fatty acids and eicosanoids. Champaign, IL: American Oil Chemists' Society, 1987: 238-240.

Oliw E, Granström E, Änggård E. The prostaglandins and essential fatty acids. In: Pace-Asciak C, Granström E, eds. New comprehensive biochemistry, Vol. 5. Prostaglandins and related substances. Amsterdam: Elsevier, 1983: 1-44.

Pollard M, Luckert PH. Effect of indomethacin on intestinal
    tumors induced in rats by the acetate derivative of dimethyl-
    nitrosamine. Science 1981;214:558-559.

Reddy BS. Dietary fat and colon cancer: effect of fish oil. In:
    Lands WEM, ed. Proc. AOCS short course on polyunsatu-
    rated fatty acids and eicosanoids. Champaign, IL: American
    Oil Chemists' Society, 1987: 233-237.

Reddy BS, Maeura Y. Tumor promotion by dietary fat in azoxy-
    methane-induced colon carcinogenesis in female F344 rats:
    influence of amount and source of dietary fat. J Natl Cancer
    Inst 1984;72:745-750.

Reddy BS, Maruyama H. Effect of dietary fish oil on azoxymeth-
    ane-induced colon carcinogenesis in male F344 rats. Cancer
    Res 1986;46:3367-3370.

Reitz RC, Borgeson CE, Pardini L, Pardini RS. Effects of dietary
    fish oil on the growth of a human mammary carcinoma in
    the athymic nude mouse and on the activity of the carnitine
    acyltransferase and the delta-9 acyl Co-A desaturase. In:
    Lands WEM, ed. Proc. AOCS short course on polyunsatu-
    rated fatty acids and eicosanoids. Champaign, IL: American
    Oil Chemists' Society, 1987: 529-533.

Roebuck BD, Yager JD Jr, Longnecker DS, Wilpone SA. Promo-
    tion by unsaturated fat of azaserine-induced pancreatic car-
    cinogenesis in the rat. Cancer Res 1981;41:3961-3966.

Stampfer MJ, Willett WC, Colditz GA, Speizer FE. Intake of
    cholesterol, fish and specific types of fat in relation to risk
    of breast cancer. In: Lands WEM, ed. Proc. AOCS short
    course on polyunsaturated fatty acids and eicosanoids.
    Champaign, IL: American Oil Chemists' Society, 1987:
    248-252.

Tannenbaum A. The genesis and growth of tumors. III. Effects
    of a high-fat diet. Cancer Res 1942;2:468-475.

Waterhouse J, Muir C, Shanmugaratnam K, et al. Cancer inci-
    dence in five continents, Vol. IV. Lyon: International
    Agency for Research on Cancer, 1982.

Watson AF, Mellanby E. Tar cancer in mice. II. The condition of
    the skin when modified by external treatment or diet, as a
    factor in influencing the cancerous reaction. Br J Exp
    Pathol 1930;11:311-322.

6
Omega-3 Fatty Acids in Growth and Development

Artemis P. Simopoulos*
International Life Sciences Institute of Research Foundation
Washington, D.C.

INTRODUCTION

There are two classes of essential polyunsaturated fatty acids: omega-6†, represented by 18:2w6, linoleic-acid (LA), and omega-3†, represented by 18:3w3, alpha-linolenic acid (LNA) (Table 1). Both LA and LNA must come from the diet because synthesis of the omega-3 and omega-6 structures has not been detected in animals. LA is universally found in the vegetable kingdom and is particularly rich in most, but not all, vegetable seeds and in the oils produced from the seeds (with coconut oil, cocoa butter, and palm oil being exceptions). LNA, on the other hand, is more restricted in nature than LA and is found in the chloroplast of green leafy plants (Table 2) and in a few vegetable oils such as linseed, rapeseed, soybean, and walnut (Table 3).

---

*Present affiliation: American Association for World Health, Washington, D.C.
†Defined by the position of the double bond closest to the methyl end of the molecule.

Table 1 EFA Metabolism Desaturation and Elongation of Omega-6 and Omega-3

Linoleate series	Linolenate series
C18:2w6 Linoleic acid	C18:3w3 Alpha-linolenic acid
Δ^6 desaturase $\rightarrow$	Δ^6 desaturase $\rightarrow$
C18:3w6 Gamma-linolenic acid	C18:4w3
$\rightarrow$	$\rightarrow$
C20:3w6 Dihomo-gamma-Linolenic Acid	C20:4w3
Δ^5 desaturase $\rightarrow$	Δ^5 desaturase $\rightarrow$
C20:4w6 Arachidonic acid	C20:5w3 Eicosapentaenoic acid
$\rightarrow$	$\rightarrow$
C22:4w6 Docosapentaenoic acid	C22:5w3 Docosapentaenoic acid
Δ^4 desaturase $\rightarrow$	Δ^4 desaturase $\rightarrow$
C22:5w6 Docosapentaenoic acid	C22:6w3 Docosahexaenoic acid

Table 2   Fatty Acid Content of Plants[a]

Fatty acid	Purslane	Spinach	Buttercrunch lettuce	Red leaf lettuce	Mustard
14:0	0.16	0.03	0.01	0.03	0.02
16:0	0.81	0.16	0.07	0.10	0.13
18:0	0.20	0.01	0.02	0.01	0.02
18:1w9	0.43	0.04	0.03	0.01	0.01
18:2w6	0.89	0.14	0.10	0.12	0.12
18:3w3	4.05	0.89	0.26	0.31	0.48
20:5w3	0.01	0.00	0.00	0.00	0.00
22:6w3	0.00	0.00	0.001	0.002	0.001
Other	1.95	0.43	0.11	0.12	0.32
Total fatty acid content	8.50	1.70	0.601	0.702	1.101

[a]mg/g of wet weight.
Source: Simopoulos and Salem, 1986.

Table 3   Terrestrial Sources of Omega-3 Fatty Acids

Oils[a]	18:3 (q)
Linseed oil	53.3
Rapeseed oil (canola)	11.1
Rice bran oil	1.6
Soybean oil	6.8
Tomatoseed oil	2.3
Walnut oil	10.4
Wheat germ oil	6.9

[a]100 g edible portion, raw.
Source: Provisional table on the content of omega-3 fatty acids and other fat components in selected foods, U.S. Department of Agriculture, Washington, DC, February 1986.

Although food selection patterns of land mammals vary and
the diet of some herbivorous species may include more leaf or
more seed material, most mammals will obtain LA and LNA from
their food. After absorption the liver metabolizes these parent
vegetable acids, increasing the chain length and degree of unsaturation by adding extra double bonds close to the carboxyl group.
This process results in two families of fatty acids with 20 and 22
carbons and four, five, or six double bonds (Table 1).

Both LA and LNA and their long-chain derivatives are important components of animal and plant membranes, although
membrane functions are not yet understood at the molecular level
for either the omega-3 or the omega-6 series of fatty acids.

Animals and humans, with the exception of carnivores
such as lions and cats, can convert LNA to eicosapentaenoic acid
(20:5w3 or EPA) and docosahexaenoic acid (22:6w3 or DHA),
but this conversion is slow in humans (Sanders and Younger,
1981). EPA and DHA can be obtained by carnivores directly from
the flesh of other mammals. EPA and DHA are found in membrane phospholipids of platelets, neutrophils, monocytes, endothelial cells, and practically all cells of individuals who are ingesting omega-3 fatty acids.

Human leukocytes and human and rat liver cells elongate
and desaturate LNA to EPA and DHA (de Gomez Dumm and
Brenner, 1975). There is competition between omega-3 and
omega-6 fatty acids for the desaturation enzymes. However, both
delta-4 and delta-6 desaturates prefer omega-3 to omega-6 fatty
acids (de Gomez Dumm and Brenner, 1975; Hague and Christoffersen, 1984). There is some evidence that the delta-6 desaturation values decrease with age (de Gomez Dumm and Brenner,
1975). Studies with suspended rat hepatocytes have shown that
retroconversion of DHA and arachidonic acid (22:4w6 or AA)
also occurs to shorter-chain fatty acids, brought about by peroxisomal beta-oxidation (Hague and Christoffersen, 1986).

LA is the precursor of AA and the predominant polyunsaturated fatty acid (PUFA) in the Western diet. AA is the precursor of the 2-series of prostanoids (prostaglandins and thromboxanes) and of leukotrienes of the 4-series. EPA and DHA are
precursors of the prostanoids of the 3-series and leukotrienes of

the 5-series (Needleman et al., 1979; Weber et al., 1986). There is functional antagonism between the prostaglandins and leukotrienes derived from EPA and those derived from AA (Weber et al., 1986; Needleman et al., 1979).

In mammals and birds, the omega-3 fatty acids are distributed among lipid classes rather selectively. LNA is found in triglycerides, in cholesteryl esters, and in very small amounts of phospholipids. EPA is found in cholesteryl esters, triglycerides, and phospholipids. DHA is found mostly in phospholipids. In the mammals, including human beings, the cerebral cortex (O'Brien and Sampson, 1965), retina (Anderson, 1970), testis, and sperm (Poulos et al., 1975) are particularly rich in DHA. DHA is one of the most abundant components of the brain's structural lipids. DHA can be derived only from direct ingestion or by synthesis from dietary LNA.

The phospholipid class and fatty acid composition and cholesterol content of biomembranes are critical determinants of membrane physical properties and have been shown to influence a wide variety of membrane-dependent functions, such as integral enzyme activity, membrane transport, and receptor function. The ability to alter membrane lipid composition and function in vivo by diet, even when EFA are adequately supplied, demonstrates the importance of diet in growth and metabolism (Galli et al., 1971a).

Svennerholm in 1968 reported on the distribution and fatty acid composition of phosphoglycerides in normal human brain from the early fetal stage to old age. He found a lipid-specific pattern for each of the four major phosphoglycerides [phosphatidylethanolamine (PE), phosphatidylcholine (PC), phosphatidylserine (PS), and phosphatidylinositol (PI)] and a tissue-specific pattern. The phospholipids of cerebral white matter contained more monoenoic acid but much less PUFA than those of cerebral cortex. There was also an age-dependent fatty acid pattern. With increasing age, the concentration of the fatty acids of the linoleate family decreased, while that of the linolenate family increased. In 1972, Crawford and Sinclair showed that in 24 mammalian species both the linoleic and linolenic series are structural components of brain, liver, and other tissues and that the ratio is species and tissue specific.

ALPHA-LINOLENIC ACID METABOLISM TO ITS LONGER-CHAIN FATTY ACIDS

In order to understand the effects of omega-3 fatty acids on growth and development, it is essential that we understand the metabolism of LNA to its longer-chain fatty acids, particularly EPA and DHA.

Over the past 10 years, research on the health effects of omega-3 fatty acids has been carried out predominantly with omega-3 fatty acids from aquatic sources—specifically, fish and fish oils that are rich in EPA and DHA (Simopoulos et al., 1986). However, in parallel with the large number of studies involving fish and fish oils, a number of investigators have carried out studies using linseed oil produced from flaxseed (a terrestrial source of omega-3 fatty acids rich in LNA) (Mest et al., 1983; Adam et al., 1984; Budowski et al., 1984; Sanders and Younger, 1981). These studies indicate that LNA influences prostaglandin metabolism and platelet aggregation as does EPA, but to a lesser extent.

The elongation and desaturation rate of LNA to EPA and DHA in humans has been the subject of considerable interest and debate (Johnston and Fritsche, 1986; Salem et al., 1986). Such conversion has been shown to occur in human fibroblasts (Aeberhard et al., 1978) and retinoblastoma cells (Hyman and Spector, 1981) in vitro. Mest et al. (1983) found that ingestion of 30 ml/day of linseed oil by human beings led to increases of 328% and 182% in EPA and DHA, respectively, in serum phospholipids. Berry and Hirsch (1986) observed a correlation between adipose tissue LNA content and systolic, diastolic, and composite mean arterial blood pressure. An absolute increase of 1% in adipose tissue LNA was associated with a decrease in blood pressure of 5 mm Hg. Since adipose tissue fatty acid content reflects dietary fat intake (Hirsch et al., 1960), these results indicate that the long-term intake of LNA or its metabolites may influence blood pressure. In addition, it has been shown that incubation of Ehrlich ascites tumor cells with LNA increased the cellular content of this fatty acid along with a concomitant increase in membrane fluidity (King and Spector, 1978).

Adam et al. (1984) carried out studies in normal volunteers using linseed oil and showed that prostaglandin production was depressed linearly with increasing intakes of linseed oil. Similarly, Budowski et al. in 1984 were able to show decreased platelet aggregability after ingestion of linseed oil in two subjects. A very interesting study of 1 year's duration was carried out by Renaud et al. in 1980 in a group of French farmers. A group of families previously on a high intake of saturated fatty acids was encouraged to change their diet and replace butter with oil and margarine rich in LNA and LA. After 1 year on the dietary regimen, the dietary content of LNA increased from 1.2% to 3.6% of the total dietary fatty acids. This led to a significant but moderate increase in the content of EPA, in both plasma and platelets, which led to prolonged coagulation time and decreased aggregation of platelets. There were no changes in plasma total cholesterol. Although the changes in EPA were moderate, they led to marked changes in platelet behavior. In a subsequent paper, Renaud and Nordoy (1983) stated that "alpha-linolenic acid is elongated and desaturated to EPA in man. Even if the absolute concentration of EPA in platelet phospholipids is low, the changes are associated with striking changes in platelet behavior. This may indicate that minor changes in tissue fatty acid composition in man may be most significant in the context of thrombosis prevention." Renaud et al. (1986) reported on the influence of long-term diet modification on platelet function and composition in Moselle farmers, which confirmed their previous findings and conclusions.

Although a number of studies indicate that human beings can form EPA and DHA from LNA, a study carried out in diabetics fed linseed oil failed to show an increase in the EPA level of plasma phospholipids. This finding suggests that diabetics may have a metabolic abnormality in the elongation and desaturation system for fatty acids (Honigmann et al., 1982).

Sanders and Younger in 1981 studied the effect of dietary supplements of LNA, EPA, and DHA on the fatty acid composi-

Table 4   Breast-Milk Fatty Acids in Vegans and Omnivore
Controls[a]

Methyl esters	Vegans (range)	Controls (range)
12:0	21-76	19-51
14:0	50-118	68-90
16:0	139-204	246-293
18:0	37-66	84-123
16:1	11-15	25-46
18:1	277-383	331-383
18:2w6	202-397	56-91
18:3w3	9-20	7-9
20:2w6	4.3-7.2	1.4-2.6
20:3w6	1.2-4.6	2.0-2.6
20:4w6	2.1-12.1	3.4-9.2
22:4w6	0.4-2.7	0.4-1.2
22:5w6	0.1-2.0	0.1-5.1
20:4w3	0.2-0.4	0.4-1.5
20:5w3	0.2-0.8	0.4-3.6
22:5w3	0.5-6.6	2.0-13.3
22:6w3	0.2-5.5	2.4-12.2

[a]Mean values expressed as mg/g total methyl esters detected for four vegans
and four omnivore controls.
Source: Adapted from Sanders et al., 1978.

tion of platelets and plasma choline phosphoglycerides in vegans
and omnivores. They found that the supplement of LNA led to
an increase in EPA but was less effective than the supplement of
EPA and DHA, indicating that the conversion of LNA to EPA
occurs but is slow.

Recent experimental studies in the rat comparing the effects
of LNA, EPA, and DHA on AA metabolism indicate that the levels
of 6-keto-PGF$_{1a}$ as determined by radioimmunoassay were reduced by dietary LNA or fish oils in a dose-dependent fashion
(Boudreau et al., 1987). The authors concluded that the reductions in 6-keto-PFG$_{1a}$ and AA were more pronounced in groups

receiving fish oil than in those receiving LNA. These results indicate that longer-chain omega-3 fatty acids rich in fish oil are more effective in reducing levels of AA and their metabolites than LNA. However, since LNA is the major PUFA of chloroplast lipids, green vegetables can be used as an alternative and/or additional dietary source of omega-3 fatty acids. It should be pointed out that vegan mother's milk contains LNA, EPA, and DHA, but a lesser amount than the milk of omnivores (Table 4) (Sanders et al., 1978). Apparently, adequate amounts of EPA and DHA are formed from LNA to sustain growth and development of the infants of vegan mothers.

ESSENTIAL FATTY ACID DEFICIENCY

Holman (1970) credits Aron in 1918 as the first to suggest that fats have nutritional functions other than provision of food energy. In 1919, Von Groer reported on two infants who were on skim milk diets for 9 months and had retarded growth, poor appetite, and possible respiratory infections. After their diets were supplemented with EFA for several months, these infants were found to be healthy, with a normal growth rate and weight gain.

In 1929, Burr and Burr were the first to produce a fat-free experimental diet and showed that fat-free diets will not support reproduction, and experimental diets deficient in fatty acids are associated with clinical symptoms such as skin rash, retardation of brain growth, incomplete brain cell division, and a high neonatal mortality in second-generation rat pups.

Further work by Burr and Burr (1930) showed that adding fatty acids to the diet, especially LA, restored the effects caused by the fat-free diet in the deprived animals. Thus, they coined the term "essential fatty acids" (EFA). The EFAs discovered by Burr and Burr included both LA and LNA. Whereas healthy skin and successful growth, reproduction, and lactation were obtained in mammals fed LA as the only source of EFA, LNA was found to permit growth but was unable to prevent the skin lesions of EFA deficiency or support reproduction.

Holt et al. in 1935 reported on one of the most significant studies on EFA deficiency in infants. Holt and colleagues fed three infants low-fat diets. The infants were closely monitored. One of them developed bronchitis and eczema. These symptoms disappeared when fat was added to the diet and reappeared on a low-fat diet. Many other studies since then have confirmed these findings. In 1958, Hansen et al. showed that LA was required by human beings; signs and symptoms of EFA deficiency could be produced in a month's time by feeding *healthy* infants skim milk as the only calorie source.

In 1960, Holman introduced the concept of the trienoic/tetraenoic acid ratio as an indicator of the severity of EFA deficiency in rats and later demonstrated its applicability to other species. A ratio of 0.4 or greater was considered indicative of EFA deficiency. Holman in 1970 suggested that the upper limit of normality is a ratio of 0.2 for humans.

In a series of papers from 1960 to 1970, Holman estimated that 1-2% of total caloric intake is required as LA to avoid the biochemical and clinical signs of EFA deficiency in human beings. EFA deficiency has been reported in both children and adults with cystic fibrosis, malabsorption, and bowel resection.

Despite all the knowledge accumulated from animal research, EFA deficiency in humans was rarely reported until the introduction of total parenteral nutrition (TPN). Since the introduction of long-term TPN, many cases of EFA deficiency have been reported occurring throughout the lifecycle, from low-birth-weight infants to the elderly (Friedman and Frolich, 1979; Holman et al., 1982; Martinez and Ballabriga, 1987; Bjerve et al., 1987). Continuous fat-free TPN inhibits the mobilization of the body's fat stores and therefore sets the stage for the development of EFA deficiency.

Galli et al. (1971b) and Paoletti and Galli (1972) concluded that dietary EFA deficiency affected the developing central nervous system and that the nutritional stress may be of comparable gravity to that due to protein and/or calorie malnutrition. In LNA deficiency 22:5w6 increased and LNA supplementation raised the proportion of 22:6w3 in brain glycerophosphatides.

Galli et al. (1974) proposed to consider the ratio of 22:5w6/22:6w3 in tissue lipids as an index of relative LNA deficiency.

Today, it is still not certain what metabolic functions EFAs perform in correcting EFA deficiency. Two main areas in which omega-6 and omega-3 fatty acids function are in prostaglandin metabolism and as structural lipids that are components of cell membranes. PUFAs also have a role in the formation of membrane phospholipids and in lipid transport.

OMEGA-3 FATTY ACID DEFICIENCY AND DEVELOPMENT: ANIMAL STUDIES

Over the past 25 years, studies on the role of omega-3 fatty acids, particularly DHA, in the rat and the rhesus monkey have indicated that dietary restriction of omega-3 fatty acids during pregnancy and lactation interferes with normal visual function and may even impair learning ability in the offspring (Walker, 1967; Benolken et al., 1973; Fiennes et al., 1973; Lamptey and Walker, 1976; Neuringer et al., 1984).

For many years, studies on EFA were dominated by studies on the effects of the omega-6 family in growth and development, despite the fact that since the identification of the fatty acids for EFA "activity," LNA had been included in the list of active substances. There are a number of reasons for not focusing on omega-3 fatty acids. First, following the discovery of EFA deficiency and its effects in animals, it was common practice not to distinguish between the acids of the LA and LNA series, and to assume that the vegetable oils contained only linoleic whereas most oils contain small amounts of linolenic acid (Hilditch and Williams, 1964). Second, it was difficult to produce DHA deficiency because brain fatty acid patterns are established early in life and are relatively stable; nutritional experiments employing weanling animals were somewhat ineffective in lowering the 22:6w3 content of the brain. As a result, it was difficult to show signs of omega-3 fatty acid deficiency. It was, therefore, necessary to carry out experiments in animals that had been on omega-3-deficient diets for more than one generation. This was accomplished by

Walker (1967), who demonstrated that restriction of dietary LNA in the maternal diet of rats was reflected in a lowering of the 22: 6w3 in the brain lipids of the pups at birth. Thus, he was able to produce DHA deficiency in the rat for the first time. However, even low levels of linolenate in the diet of the lactating dam resulted in rapid accumulation of the DHA in the brain. This marked affinity of brain lipids for DHA raised the possibility of a functional requirement for linolenic acid.

Another major advance was the discovery by Benolken et al. (1973) on the relationship between dietary LNA and the electro-retinogram (ERG) response in the rat.

Wheeler et al. (1975) measured ERGs in rats as a function of dietary supplements of purified ethyl esters of LNA, LA, and oleic acids. PUFAs derived from LNA and LA appear to be important functional components of photoreceptor cell membranes. LNA affected the ERG amplitudes to a greater extent than LA. The authors concluded that "the electrical response of photoreceptor cell membranes appears to be a function of the position of the double bonds as well as a function of the total number of double bonds in fatty acids supplements." These findings indicate a selective functional role in the visual system for omega-3 fatty acids and suggest that the observed electrical alterations are associated with fatty acid substitutions in the plasma membrane.

Vertebrate photoreceptor cells consist of an inner and an outer segment. The inner segment of the rod cell contains a variety of membrane systems, such as mitochondrial, ribosomal, plasma, and nuclear membranes. The rod outer segments (ROS) are characterized by a stacked array of many hundreds of disk membranes which are enclosed by a plasma membrane. The visual pigment rhodospin accounts for 80-90% of ROS membrane-bound protein and phospholipids account for 80-85% of the total ROS membrane lipid. Phospholipids are required for both the stability and regenerability of rhodopsin and, on the average, each rhodopsin molecule of rat ROS is associated with 60-65 phospholipid molecules. DHA is the dominant PUFA of the phospholipids of vertebrate ROS membranes (Wheeler et al., 1975).

The studies by Walker (1967) and Wheeler et al. (1975) were very important and set the stage as standards upon which further studies on the role of omega-3 fatty acids on retina and brain function were based. Walker's study showed that DHA deficiency could be developed by using omega-3-deficient diets during pregnancy and postnatally. Wheeler et al. established that DHA deficiency in retina could be reflected by measuring ERG amplitude changes.

The knowledge obtained from the studies of Walker (1967) and Wheeler et al. (1975) led Lamptey and Walker (1976) to undertake a study in which safflower oil, which has a high linoleic/linolenic acid ratio, was included in the diet of female rats prior to mating and during pregnancy and lactation. Progeny were weaned to the same diet and their physical, neuromotor, and neurophysiological development assessed in relation to pups from dams fed a diet containing soybean oil. Brain lipids were compared in the two groups of animals. Reviewing this study today brings excitement and admiration for the work of these investigators. Their interpretation of the results of their monumental study follows:

> Perhaps the most significant observation in the current study was the apparent lower proficiency in learning in the mature rats raised on the safflower oil diet. Of interest in this respect was the performance of rats raised on a corn oil-containing diet in another study. In these latter animals, the 22:6w3 content of the brain ethanolamine glycerophosphatide was intermediate between those of the two groups in the current study; performance in the Y-maze test was also intermediate between safflower and soybean oil-fed groups (Witting et al., 1961). Animals fed a linoleate- and linolenate-deficient diet (hydrogenated coconut oil) exhibited Y-maze performances greatly inferior to the three groups referred to above. A similar impairment in learning ability by essential fatty acid-deficient rats has been reported (Paoletti and Galli, 1972).
> Although the data suggest a learning deficit may be due to the lack of linolenic acid in the safflower oil-fed rats, the nature of the test employed must be kept in mind. This was

not a simple assessment of the animal's ability to learn but
also involved its ability to discriminate between the white
and black end-goal boxes. Benolken et al. (1973) have associated linolenic acid metabolites with the electrical responses
of the photoreceptor membranes of the eye and the possibility that results obtained in the current study reflect an impairment in the visual processes of the rat cannot be dis-
counted.

It is highly speculative to associate chemical aspects in
the structural lipids of the brain with specific changes in be-
havioral patterns particularly on the basis of a single study.
In the present study, low dietary levels of linolenic acid were
manifest in low levels of the w-3 acids, particularly 22:6w3,
in the brain ethanolamine glycerophosphatides. Evidence
was obtained for a lower proficiency in a simple discrimina-
tion-learning task and possibly of a reduction in exploratory
activity in these animals. Further evidence is required to
substantiate the thesis that 22:6w3 performs a specific function in brain lipids not shared by the w-6 polyunsaturated
acids thus making linolenic acid a dietary essential. Confirm-
ation of this observation would support existing evidence for
the essentiality of the w-3 acids based on the growth response
in monkeys (Fiennes et al., 1973) and the neurophysiological
function reported in the photoreceptor membranes (Benolken et al., 1973).

The first experimental evidence of LNA deficiency or LNA requirement in primates (capuchins) was reported by Fiennes et al.
in 1973. Despite the fact that the capuchins received adequate
amounts of LA, they suffered from symptoms closely resembling
those of EFA, which were improved by the addition of linseed
oil to the diet (55.7% LNA). Of interest is the fact that although
the capuchins were on a purified diet (24-28 months) containing
very little LNA, the liver and red blood cells PE still contained
about 6% of their fatty acids as LNA metabolites, mostly DHA.
This finding is similar to the results of linoleic-acid-deficient diets
fed to rats, where it has been found difficult to deplete their tissues of AA (Walker, 1967). The red blood cell fatty acids of the
capuchins had the characteristic profile already known from the

studies in rats fed a diet high in LA and poor in LNA (Galli et al., 1971b); namely, elevated levels of 22:4w6 and 22:5w6 and low levels of 22:6w3. In discussing their findings, Fiennes et al. state:

> The main question raised by our observations centers on the essentiality of linolenic acid. It has been known for some time that animals cannot synthesize linoleic and linolenic acids (Burr and Burr, 1930). Most of the work of EFA has been done in the laboratory rat which has a short breeding interval and life span. In the rat skin symptoms associated with EFA deficiency can apparently be cured by corn oil and it has been assumed that linolenic acid is unnecessary for rats and other species including man (Witting, 1970). Species specificity exists in the fatty acids of structural lipids and it has already been established that the fatty acids on the structural lipids of large and small mammals are quite different (Crawford and Sinclair, 1972); therefore, the requirements are likely to be different.
>
> Capuchins eat a diet in the natural habitat which includes insect food and a variety of vegetable material, such as nuts, fruit and leaf shoots. Their intake of EFA will certainly not be confined to those of the linoleic series, because green leaf material, vegetation growing points, small insects and animals would provide significant quantities of linolenic acid and its derivatives.
>
> These results indicate that a linolenic acid deficiency was induced in the capuchins, although further investigations are required on both the biochemistry and pathology.

Because primates are closer to human beings in retinal structure and visual function, Neuringer et al. (1984) carried out a series of studies in the infant rhesus monkey (*Macaca mulatta*) that had been DHA deficient during gestation and postnatally. These investigators demonstrated that maternal omega-3 fatty acid deprivation led to abnormally low levels of DHA in the tissues of the near-term fetus and newborn infant; and that vulnerability to dietary omega-3 fatty acid deprivation appeared to be even greater after birth. In 1986, Neuringer et al. reported on the biochemical and functional effects of prenatal and postnatal omega-3 fatty acid deficiency on retina and brain in the DHA-deprived rhesus monkeys during pregnancy and lactation, up to 22 months of age. The control monkeys showed an increase in the 22:6w3 in the central cortex and retina, about double that at birth. The deficient monkeys, on the other hand, failed to increase retina and brain DHA at 22 months (the 22:6w3 of PE was one-half of the control values in the retinal and one-fourth in cerebral cortex). As was the case with rat studies (Galli et al., 1971b) and capuchin studies (Fiennes et al., 1973), the low levels of 22:6w3 in the deficient animals' tissues were accompanied by a compensatory increase in longer-chain omega-6 fatty acids, particularly 22:5w6. Subnormal visual acuity at 4-12 weeks of age and prolonged recovery time of the dark-adapted electroretinogram after a saturating light flash were noted in the deficient monkeys. The authors point out:

> The fatty acid composition of the cerebral cortex described here for control newborn and juvenile rhesus monkeys are very similar to those reported by Svennerhold (1968) for human newborns and adolescents, respectively. However, the brain and retina of human infants are less developed at birth than those of rhesus monkeys (Cheek, 1975), so that human infants might be even more vulnerable to postnatal dietary deprivation of w3 fatty acids.
>   They concluded:
> Our findings provide evidence that dietary w3 fatty acids are essential for normal prenatal and postnatal development of the retina and brain. Further research will be required to determine the relative contributions of prenatal versus postnatal deprivation to the observed functional deficits and to determine the degree to which the biochemical and functional effects of w3 fatty acid deficiency are reversible.

Rotstein et al. (1987) carried out studies on the effects of aging on the composition and metabolism of DHA-containing lipids of the retina in the rat. These investigators studied the effects of aging on the compositional and metabolic aspects of retinal phospholipids. They showed that the levels of DHA as well as of other w-3 hexaenoic acids were decreased in retinal glycerophospholipids of aging rats, especially in those containing choline

and serine. In comparing the in vitro labeling of retinal lipids with
[2-^{3}H] glycerol and [1-^{14}C] DHA in young and aged animals, the
authors found that most retinal lipid classes incorporate DHA, particularly when the DHA content is decreased, and that this incorporation is further stimulated by aging. Therefore, the decrease in
the DHA content of retinal phospholipids is not due to an impaired activity of the enzymes involved in the synthesis and turn-
over of phospholipids, but to a decreased availability of DHA to
the retina. In fact, retinas of aging rats had a greater affinity for
DHA than those of younger rats. The authors state:

> The results allow us to conclude that the levels of 22:6-con-
> taining species of lipids are decreased during aging simply
> because there is less 22:6 available in the retina, since when
> the fatty acid is provided the enzymes work to attain, and
> even surpass, their fullest capacity.

Since the levels of the w-3 pentaenoic acids in retinal lipids
were much less affected by aging than the w-3 hexaenoic acids,
these results indicate that there was no defect in the availability
of 18:3w3 or its metabolic products up to 22:5w3. Furthermore,
the findings indicate an important difference between the effects
of aging and EFA deficiency on the retina. With 18:2w6 (linoleic
acid) deficiency, 20:4w6 is decreased in tissue lipids and is replaced by 22:3w9 (from oleic acid). During 18:3w3 (linolenic
acid) deficiency 22:6w3 decreases in lipids and is replaced by
22:5w6 (from linoleic acid). None of these compensatory mechanisms were shown to occur in the retina of the aging rat. Both
22:5w6 and 22:6w3 fatty acids require delta$_4$ desaturase for their
synthesis. This strongly suggests that, rather than a decreased
availability of 18:3w3 (and 18:2w6) in the retina, an impairment
of the delta$_4$ desaturase enzyme system is probably responsible
for the decreased levels of 22:6w3 (and 22:5w6) observed in
retinal lipids as a consequence of aging.

In view of the fact that DHA is required for normal function
of photoreceptors in rats and primates, it is quite possible that a
decrease in DHA plays an important role in visual impairments
that accompany old age. One could speculate that an adequate

dietary supply of DHA, rather than LNA, might influence the development of visual impairments and even improve visual function in the elderly.

OMEGA-3 FATTY ACID DEFICIENCY AND DEVELOPMENT: HUMAN STUDIES

Pregnancy

Over the past 50 years, the influence of maternal nutrition on fetal growth has been extensively studied in the context of protein-calorie malnutrition. As noted earlier, the role of EFA in pregnancy has been examined only over the past 15 years in animals and only very recently in human beings.

In 1985, Olsen and Joensen reported that the birth weights in the Faroe Islands were higher than those in Denmark; in fact, they were higher than in 33 other countries. The Faroe Islands are located between Norway and Iceland. The diet of the Faroese is high in fish, higher than in Denmark. In view of the fact that dietary omega-3 PUFAs influence the fatty acid composition of tissues and cell membranes and are incorporated into the red cell membrane phospholipids, Olsen et al. (1986) determined the total omega-3 PUFAs in erythrocyte phosphatidylethanolamine in pregnant Faroese women and compared it to that of a Danish population and a Canadian population (previous studies had shown the values for Canadians to be representative of populations on the usual Western diet). The comparisons are striking. The omega-3 PUFAs (expressed as a percent of the total amount of fatty acids present, mean $\pm$ SD) were 15.2 ± 27 for the pregnant Faroese women vs. 9.7 for the pregnant Canadian controls. The length of gestation was 40.3 ± 1.7 for the Faroese vs. 39.7 ± 1.8 for the Danish pregnant women ($p = 0.05$), and the average birth weight of infants or primiparas was 194 g higher for the Faroese. The authors hypothesized that the higher dietary omega-3 intake influenced endogenous prostaglandin metabolism. They suggest that dietary omega-3 inhibited the production of the dienoic prostaglandins, primarily PGF_{2a} and PGE_2 (the prostaglandins that mediate uterine contraction and the ripening of the cervix and lead to labor and delivery.

These human epidemiological findings indicating an increase in the birth weight with an increase in fish intake and an increase in the percent of total omega-3 fatty acids in red cell phosphatidylethanolamine suggest that ingestion of fish and fish oil may play an important role in length of gestation. Certainly, these observations ought to be further investigated since the prevention of prematurity is one of the most critical issues to be overcome in perinatal medicine. Prematurity and low birth weight are associated with high risk of handicaps related to the brain and nervous system.

Crawford et al. (1981) calculated the EFA requirements for pregnancy in terms of LA and LNA to be between 600 and 650 g, or about 1% of the nonpregnant woman's dietary energy, and another 0.5% of energy for AA and DHA.

Placental Fatty Acid Metabolism

Crawford et al. (1981) examined fatty acids in phosphatidylcholine (PC) and phosphatidylethanolamine (PE) in maternal plasma, fetal cord blood, fetal liver, and brain from the human fetus at midterm abortion. The concentration of LA decreased and that of AA increased progressively in the PC and PE from maternal liver to cord blood, to fetal liver, and finally to fetal brain. The same progression was observed with LNA. These investigators termed the sequence a process of "biomagnification." This process is responsible for the high content of AA and DHA, originating from linoleic and linolenic acids, respectively, in the brain. Thus, a concentration gradient is established across the placenta by preferential transfer of DHA and AA to the fetal side of the placenta.

Human placenta in vitro synthesizes AA (Zimmerman et al., 1979). In the in vitro system used, there was simultaneous accumulation of both omega-6 and omega-3 chain elongation-desaturation products.

Fetal Development

Rapid synthesis of brain tissue occurs during the third trimester of human development, in association with increasing neuromotor activity. Cell size, type, and number increase, requiring de novo synthesis of structural lipids by the developing fetus. Martinez and associates (1974 and 1978) and Clandinin and associates (1980) have shown that in the human infant, DHA accumulates in the brain during the last trimester. Clandinin et al. (1980) studied the intrauterine fatty acid accretion rates in human brain and reported:

> Quantitative fatty acid analysis of the brain throughout this period of organogenesis indicates that tissue accretion of saturated and w-9 fatty acids, as well as total fatty acid content, paralleled increases in whole brain weight. Levels of linoleic and linolenic acids were consistently low in brain during the last trimester of development, while marked substantial accretion of long chain desaturation products, arachidonic and docosahexaenoic acids occurred. Accretion of individual fatty acids of cerebellum also reflected changes in tissue total fatty acid content, with exception of the levels of linolenic acid and its chain elongation products present in cerebellum during the last trimester.

More recently, Martinez and Ballabriga (1987) studied the developmental changes in the fatty acid composition of the main phosphoglycerides of the human liver and brain during the second half of gestation. Eighteen newborn infants with gestational ages between 20 and 44 weeks were divided into three groups according to their gestational age: A very immature group ranged from 20 to 25 weeks, an immature group from 28 to 31 weeks, and a full-term group 37 weeks and over. The data indicated that the main developmental changes in the brain were an increase in DHA at the end of gestation and a decrease in 18:1w9 (oleic acid) and AA in PE. These data confirmed their previous findings (Martinez et al., 1974; Martinez and Ballabriga, 1978). Similar changes were noted in the liver. There was a marked increase in DHA in both PE and PC at the end of gestation and a linear decrease in 18:1w9 and AA in PE and PC. These changes were significant at the 0.001

Table 5   Fatty Acids in Ethanolamine Phosphoglycerides in
Human Liver and Brain: Effect of Development

Organ	20-25 weeks ($n = 6$)	28-31 weeks ($n = 6$)	37 weeks ($n = 6$)
Human liver			
22:5w3	0.3 ± 0.11	0.3 ± 0.06	0.6 ± 0.21
22:6w3	11.5 ± 1.05	10.6 ± 0.96	17.7 ± 3.50
w3/w6	0.31 ± 0.04	0.29 ± 0.03	0.60 ± 0.16
Human brain			
22:5w3	0.3 ± 0.05	0.3 ± 0.05	0.5 ± 0.21
22:6w3	15.3 ± 0.58	13.8 ± 1.09	18.9 ± 1.06
w3/w6	0.41 ± 0.02	0.36 ± 0.03	0.50 ± 0.06

Source: Adapted from Martinez and Ballabriga, 1987.

level in both the brain and liver. Thus, a neonate born prior to 37
weeks has much lower amounts of DHA in brain and liver and, unless it is supplied in the diet, is at risk of becoming deficient in
DHA (Table 5).

Human Milk and Infant Feeding

Crawford et al. (1973) analyzed 32 samples of human milk and
found a mean 18:2w6 content of 8.5% and much smaller amounts
of 20:2w6, 20:3w6, 20:4w6, 22:3w6, and 22:4w6. From the w-3
family there was 18:3w3, 20:5w3, 22:5w3, and 22:6w3. Crawford et al. recommended that all of these fatty acids ought to be
considered essential, because they can be classified as structural
lipids in the human brain. They argued that, from an evolutionary
point of view, the long-chain polyunsaturates are there for a reason, and they would not be present in human milk unless there
was a function for the 18:2w6 and 18:3w3 and their long-chain
metabolic products. The authors concluded that the inclusion of
a broad spectrum of long-chain PUFAs in infant formula instead
of a single acid, 18:2w6, may be desirable for optimum development.

Table 6 Fatty Acid Composition of Human Milk and Formulas
(Molar Percent)

Fatty acid[a]	Human milk ($n = 11$)	Portagen[b]	Enfamil Premature	Similac Special Care
8:0	0.35 ± 0.00	60	24.5	24.1
10:0	1.39 ± 0.14	24	14.1	17.7
12:0	6.99 ± 0.70	0.42	12.2	14.9
14:0	7.96 ± 0.88	Trace	4.7	5.8
16:0	19.82 ± 0.37	0.19	7.5	6.8
16:1	3.20 ± 0.21		0.1	0.2
18:0	5.91 ± 0.3	0.47	1.7	2.3
18:1	34.82 ± 1.4	4.1	12.4	10.0
18:2n6	16.00 ± 1.3	8.1	22.4	17.4
18:3n3	0.62 ± 0.04	Trace	0.6	0.9
20:1	1.10 ± 0.2		0.3	0.1
20:2n6	0.61 ± 0.1			
20:3n6	0.42 ± 0.04			
20:4n6	0.59 ± 0.04			
20.5n3	0.03 ± 0.00			
22:1	0.10 ± 0.00			
22:4n6	0.21 ± 0.00			
22:5n6	0.22 ± 0.00			
22:5n3	0.09 ± 0.03			
22:6n3	0.19 ± 0.03			

[a]Values are expressed as mean ± SEM.
[b]Pediatric Products Handbook, 1983 ed., Mead Johnson Nutritional Division.
Source: Carlson et al., 1986.

Crawford et al. (1981) pointed out that in human milk, the total EFA content is approximately equivalent to the protein content, which is about 6% of the dietary energy, and they state that since "less than half of the protein amino acids are essential, the total milk EFA is greater than the total essential amino acids. These quantitative relationships are not generally appreciated because the EFA content is thought of in comparison with the total fat which is present firstly as the major energy source of milk."

Table 7 Erythrocyte Lipid Fatty Acids and Aldehydes in Vegans and Controls[a]

Methyl esters and dimethyl acetals	Vegans (range)	Controls (range)
16:0 DMA	6-35	3-22
16:0	175-245	181-264
18:0 DMA	6-32	4-35
18:0	119-195	127-175
22:0	9-36	7-25
24:0	16-57	16-45
18:1	102-185	116-160
24:1	15-106	37-87
18:2w6	79-136	52-112
20:2w6	2-18	1-13
20:3w6	1-45	4-23
20:4w6	99-155	102-149
22:4w6	29-67	9-38
22:5w6	1-25	3-11
20:5w3	Tr[b]-3	3-16
22:5w3	9-43	18-32
22:6w3	6-36	37-106

[a]Mean values expressed in mg/g total methyl esters and dimethyl acetals detected for 18 subjects of each kind.
[b]Tr denotes less than 0.5 mg/g.
Source: Adapted from Sanders et al., 1978.

The authors further indicate that "lipid provides 60% of the infant's dietary energy and 10-12% of that is the EFA component, whereas protein accounts for only 6% of the dietary energy. Furthermore, lipids play an important role in the development of the brain and the vascular system. It is quite possible that lipids-EFA may be of greater significance to early human development than protein." Yet, up to now, nutritional thinking has been dominated by concepts concerning protein and body growth. Since brain development in the human takes place during fetal life and the first two years after birth, lipid nutrition during pregnancy and lactation is of special relevance to human development. Human milk is the preferred form for infant feeding (Simopoulos and

Table 8 Erythrocyte Fatty Acids in Vegan Breast-Fed Infants and Omnivore Breast-Fed Infants[a]

Methyl esters and dimethyl acetals	Breast-fed by vegans ($n = 3$) (range)	Breast-fed by omnivores ($n = 6$) (range)
16:0 DMA	17-35	16-30
16:0	184-250	187-224
18:0 DMA	25-27	19-31
18:0	142-181	172-182
22:0	10-25	18-32
24:0	32-49	39-63
18:1	101-114	120-137
24:1	36-64	32-68
18:2w6	104-113	51-72
20:3w9		1-3
20:2w6	5-6	
20:3w6	11-15	6-11
20:4w6	121-141	114-156
22:4w6	29-40	15-33
22:5w6	4-11	1-21
20:5w3	1-2	2-12
22:5w3	9-24	12-24
22:6w3	15-25	45-72

[a]Mean values expressed in mg/g total methyl esters and dimethyl acetals detected for the number of subjects shown.
Source: Adapted from Sanders et al., 1978.

Grave, 1984). It contains both LA and LNA, as well as AA, EPA, and DHA, whereas infant formula does not contain the longer-chain EFA (Table 6). Vegan women have lower levels of the long-chain omega-3 fatty acids 22:5w3 and 22:6w3 in their erythrocytes and in their milk, and so do their breast-fed babies, than do omnivore women and their breast-fed babies (Tables 7 and 8).

Sanders and Naismith (1976) determined the long-chain PUFA content of erythrocytes from four breast-fed and eight bottle-fed babies. The fatty acids 22:5w3 and 22:6w3 were higher in erythrocytes from breast-fed babies than in those from bottle-fed babies and the acid 20:3w9 was lower in the erythrocytes of the breast-fed infants.

Studies by Clandinin and co-workers (1981a,b) have shown that human milk contains enough PUFAs to meet the needs for brain development following premature delivery. Carlson et al. (1986) studied the red blood cell phospholipids of premature infants. Their data indicate that fetal DHA is provided by maternal/placental transfer and that the DHA in human milk is adequate to supply the infant's DHA needs postnatally. Furthermore, preterm infants do not have the ability to convert LNA to DHA adequately. Clandinin et al. (1981a,b) and Crawford et al. (1972, 1976) have raised the question of the ability of the neonate to convert linoleic and linolenic acids to their long-chain polyenoates since humans appear to have a limited capacity for the Δ^4-desaturation that is responsible for the last catalytic step in the formation of 22:5w6 and 22:6w3.

Following birth there is a decrease in the red blood cell DHA in premature infants (Carlson et al., 1986). In view of the fact that the greatest amount of DHA accumulation occurs during the last trimester of pregnancy, the amount of DHA available to the premature infant assumes critical importance. Liu and co-workers (1987) carried out studies to determine whether additional DHA would be absorbed by premature infants if fish oil were incorporated into their formula. The investigators assessed DHA uptake by fatty acid analysis of plasma PE and PC. Their results indicated a rise in plasma PE DHA in infants who received fish oil DHA as a single dose of 71 mg/kg/day in a bolus, as well as those who received 11 mg/kg/day as fish oil dispersed in their formula. Infants given dispersed fish oil appeared to absorb as much or even more, despite the much lower dose. Incorporation of DHA at 11 mg/kg/day resulted in 0.2% DHA in the total dietary fatty acids in the formula, which is within the range of 0.1-0.3% found in human milk. The inclusion of 0.2% of DHA in the formula did not decrease plasma phospholipid AA and appeared to be a physiological amount that could prevent declines in membrane phospholipid DHA following preterm delivery.

Because of the evidence that DHA is one of the most abundant components of the brain structural lipids and is found in even larger amounts in the retina, Harris et al. (1984) designed a study to see whether increased dietary DHA in the mother would be reflected in a higher DHA content in human milk. They reported:

> Eight lactating women were given supplements of a fish oil concentrate rich in w-3 fatty acids, including DHA (11% of fatty acids). Six women took 5 g/day of fish oil for 28 days; five women consumed 10 g/day for 14 days; and one woman consumed 47 g/day for 8 days. Each intake level of fish oil produced significant dose-dependent increases in the DHA content of milk and plasma. Base-line DHA levels in milk were *0.01* ± 0.06% of total fatty acids. Five g/day of fish oil raised the levels to 0.5 ± 0.1% (p < 0.001); 10 g/day raised DHA levels to 0.8 ± 0.1% (p < 0.001); and 47 g/day produced DHA levels of 4.8%. The results of this study indicated that relatively low intakes of dietary DHA significantly elevated milk DHA content. This would clearly elevate the infant's DHA intake and might have implications for brain and retinal development.

The question of supplementation of infant formula, particularly for premature infants, with omega-3 fatty acids, especially DHA, is very important in view of the recent experimental evidence by Neuringer et al. (1986) which suggests that omega-3 fatty acids are essential for normal prenatal and postnatal development of the retina and brain of the rhesus monkey.

Childhood

In 1982, Holman et al. reported the first case of human LNA deficiency that was induced by long-term intravenous hyperalimentation with a preparation that was high in LA and low in LNA. The patient, a 6-year-old white girl, sustained a 22-caliber rifle wound to her abdomen that led to removal of 266 cm of small intestine, the ileocecal valve, and 34 cm of large bowel. She was maintained on TPN for many months. For a period of 7 months, she was on TPN solution high in LA and very low in LNA. The patient experienced episodes of distal numbness and paresthesia, weakness, and blurring of vision. Neurological examination was normal except for decreased peripheral vibratory sensation. Nerve conduction velocities and opthalmological examination were normal. Analysis of fatty acids of serum lipids revealed marginal linoleate deficiency but significant linolenate deficiency. Because neurological symptoms had never been reported with omega-6 deficiency in patients on TPN, omega-3 deficiency was suspected. However, it was felt that although LNA need not be essential for general growth since its major metabolite DHA is distributed preferentially in nerve and synaptic endings of the brain, it may serve a specific function in these tissues. Therefore, the regimen was changed to an emulsion that contained LNA, and the neurological symptoms disappeared. The requirement for linolenic acid was estimated to be about 0.54% of calories.

Whereas the omega-6 fatty acids were recognized as "required" for normal growth and development and a requirement was estimated for infants, older children, and adults, a requirement for omega-3 fatty acids has not yet been established in human beings. Over the past 15-20 years data from animal experiments and studies with human beings on enteral or TPN and special diets that were "low" or deficient in omega-3 fatty acids have focused attention on the importance of omega-3 acids in vision and in central nervous system function.

Aging

Whereas the apparent essential role in the development of neural tissues of young animals and the human fetus and infant is gaining acceptance, the role of omega-3 fatty acids in the elderly is only now beginning to unfold. Bjerve et al. (1987) described four patients with LNA deficiency on long-term gastric tube feeding and attempted to estimate LNA and long-chain unsaturated fatty acid requirements in human beings. They reported:

> In plasma and erythrocytes, total lipid 20:3n9 was slightly increased but total n-6 fatty acids, arachidonic acid, and dihomo-gammalinolenic acid were normal. Total n-3 fatty

acids, 18:3n3, 20:5n3, 22:5n3, and 22:6n3 were decreased in both plasma and erythrocytes. Patients had a slight but definite scaly dermatitits, which disappeared with essential fatty acid supplementation. Simultaneously levels of 18:3n3 20:5n3, 22:5n3, 22:6n3, 20:3n9, and total n-3 fatty acids became normal while 18:2n6, 20:3n6, 20:4n6, and total n-6 acids were unchanged or slightly lowered. Estimated minimal daily requirement of linolenic acid and of long-chain unsaturated n-3 acids in adults is equivalent to 0.2-0.3% and 0.1-0.2%, respectively, of total energy intake. Results suggest that conversion of linolenic acid to 22:6n3 is increased in linolenic acid deficiency.

This was the first report of omega-3 fatty acid deficiency in adults. Koletzko (1987) challenged the authors' conclusions and stated that "Bjerve et al. do not provide conclusive evidence for the existence of an n-3 fatty acid deficiency syndrome in the human adults." Bjerve (1987) responded to the challenge and provided further information on an additional patient with omega-3 fatty acid deficiency "who was treated with >99% pure ethyl-alpha-linolenate as a supplement to an otherwise unchanged per-oral feeding. Supplementing with 0.1 mL/d of ethyl-alpha-linolenate started to normalize skin changes within a week and after 14 days increased the concentration of n-3 fatty acids in red blood cells by 260%, i.e., from 24.7 to 88.1 $\mu g/10^{10}$ erythrocytes."

The responses of the skin lesions of these four patients are reminiscent of the studies by Fiennes et al. (1973), who reported skin lesions in EFA-deficient capuchin monkeys. The capuchins responded to linseed oil feeding. However, because skin lesions in EFA deficiency had always responded to supplementation with oils rich in omega-6 fatty acids, the role of omega-3 fatty acids in producing skin changes has been ignored up to now. The study of Bjerve et al. has stimulated discussion on the role of omega-3 fatty acid in improving skin lesions.

The level of omega-3 fatty acids in plasma and in red blood cells that defines the deficient state will need to be precisely defined since different investigators have used different methods and some report absolute amounts and other relative amounts (Bjerve et al., 1987).

DIETARY IMPLICATIONS

The premature infant born prior to 37 weeks' gestation appears to be particularly vulnerable to having deficient stores of DHA in the liver and brain. Since DHA deficiency is associated with reduced visual acuity in the deprived infant rhesus monkey, the need for DHA in the diet of the premature infant is receiving particular attention. As indicated in the studies by Liu et al. (1987), DHA dispersed in infant formula can be absorbed by the premature infant. These investigators have undertaken studies in premature infants with the goal of measuring development of visual acuity in supplemented and unsupplemented infants during infancy.

Similarly, the administration of omega-3 fatty acids, particularly DHA, in formula for the full-term infant requires consideration. We must also consider whether to develop infant formulas patterned after human milk in terms of the proportions of omega-3 and omega-6 fatty acids and their long-chain derivatives. Because infants fed human milk have higher plasma and blood cell DHA than those fed formula, it is essential to know if the difference between the human milk-fed and formula-fed infants is physiologically significant. With the exception of the Neuringer studies (1984 and 1986) of altered function in the rhesus monkey deprived of DHA during pregnancy and postnatally, the physiological and neurological significance of the DHA content of neural and other cellular membranes is unknown.

Both the premature infant and the retina of the aging rat have limitations in their ability to desaturate LNA to DHA. Supplying dietary fish or fish oil supplements at these two ends of the lifecycle should be carefully considered. Similarly, diabetics appear to be limited in their ability to metabolize LNA to EPA and DHA. Supplementation of rats with fish oils prevented insulin resistance induced by high-fat feeding (Storlien et al., 1987). This important finding indicates that omega-3 fatty acid in the form of fish oil supplementation might be of therapeutic or preventive value in noninsulin-dependent diabetes mellitus patients. Most importantly, Kamada et al. (1986) observed that while the levels of erythrocyte membrane fluidity were lower in patients with diabetes than in normal controls, this difference in membrane fluidity disappeared after both groups were fed 2700 mg of sarine oil daily for 8 weeks.

Particular attention needs to be paid to the composition and amount of EFA in TPN. Increased amounts of LA fed in TPN formula interfere with the metabolism of both omega-6 and omega-3 shorter-chain fatty acids to their longer-chain analogs and have led to increased levels of LA in the brain of the premature infant (Martinez and Ballabriga, 1987). Similarly, abnormal urinary prostaglandin metabolites have been reported by Friedman and Frolich (1979) in premature infants on long-term TPN that contained high levels of LA. It appeared that LA inhibited normal prostaglandin metabolism.

Furthermore Innis in 1986 studied the effects of TPN with LA-rich emulsions on tissue omega-6 and omega-3 fatty acids in the rat and concluded that "the data suggest that intravenous administration of high levels of 18:2w6 in parenteral lipid reduces desaturation/elongation of essential fatty acids but does not competitively inhibit esterification of other fatty acids into phospholipid."

In view of the fact that a number of studies indicate that LNA is converted to EPA and DHA in human beings (with the exception of the premature infant, the diabetic, and possibly the elderly), it is important to consider terrestrial sources of omega-3 fatty acids in the food supply in addition to the marine sources.

Alpha-linolenic acid, the precursor to EPA and DHA, was first isolated from hempseed in 1887 (Deuel, 1951). In plants, leaf lipids usually contain LNA, which is an important component of chloroplast membrane polar lipids. Mammals who feed on these plants convert LNA to EPA and DHA, the long-chain omega-3 fatty acids found in fish.

Wild animals and birds that feed on wild plants are very lean, with a carcass fat content of only 3.9% (Ledger, 1968), and contain about five times more polyunsaturated fat per gram than is found in domestic livestock (Crawford, 1968; Wo and Draper, 1975). Most important, 4% of the fat of wild animals contains EPA, whereas domestic beef contains very small or undetectable amounts, since cattle are fed grains rich in omega-6 fatty acids and poor in omega-3 fatty acids (Crawford et al., 1969). Deer that forage on ferns and mosses also have omega-3 fatty acids in their meat.

Over the past century, the typical Western diet has become rich in omega-6 and poor in omega-3 fatty acids (Crawford, 1968; Harris et al., 1984; Budowski and Crawford, 1985; Weber et al., 1986), The amount of fish and the level of omega-3's in the American diet was extensively discussed at a Conference on the Health Effects of Polyunsaturated Fatty Acids in Seafoods, held in June 1985 (Simopoulos et al., 1986). It was noted that in 1985, the per capita consumption of fish was 13 lb/year, which is equivalent to about one fish meal per week. Although a recommended dietary allowance has not been established, a recommendation was made to increase this amount to two to three fish meals per week.

It was further recommended that total fat intake should be 30% of total calories, with 10% being saturated, 10% monosaturated, and 10% polyunsaturated, the latter being divided equally between omega-6 and omega-3. The optimal ratio of omega-6 to omega-3 in the diet is not known; most investigators feel that it lies somewhere between 2:1 and 7:1. To that I would add that the omega-3 intake should come from both aquatic and terrestrial sources. Wild plants such as purslane have high amounts of omega-3 fatty acids (Table 2) (Simopoulos and Salem, 1986). Modern horticulturists have a challenge to produce and cultivate vegetables high in omega-3 fatty acids similar to wild plants. The new science of genetic engineering could make a major contribution in increasing the omega-3 content of plants.

Because of the apparent essential role of omega-3 fatty acids in normal growth and development, an adequate level of omega-3 fatty acids (e.g., by eating fish two to three times a week) should be included in the diet of pregnant and lactating women. Some infant formulas do contain omega-3 fatty acids, in the form of soybean oil, and the inclusion of DHA in the formula for the premature infant should be further investigated.

Table 9 Relative Content of Omega-3 Fatty Acids and Cholesterol in Fish

Species	% Oil in flesh[a]	% Omega-3 fatty acids in oil[a,b]	% Omega-3 fatty acids in flesh[c]	% Cholesterol in flesh[d]
Haddock	00.5	39.6	0.198	.060
Snapper	01.1	23.0	0.253	.040
Tuna, canned	01.0	30.0	0.300	.063
Shrimp	01.1	28.5	0.314	.180
Cod, Atlantic	00.7	45.9	0.321	.050
Pollock	00.8	48.4	0.387	.071
Sole, lemon	01.4	31.0	0.434	.050
Ocean perch	02.0	22.0	0.440	.050
Flounder	01.3	35.0	0.455	.050
Squid	01.0	53.3	0.533	.241
Mullet	03.0	19.1	0.573	.021
Halibut	02.0	36.0	0.720	.050
Shad	02.8	26.1	0.731	.038

Whiting, Pacific	03.0	33.3	0.999	.066
Swordfish	04.4	25.7	1.131	.057
Trout, rainbow	07.0	17.6	1.232	.050
Tuna, raw	05.1	30.0	1.530	.046
Whitefish, lake	07.0	22.2	1.554	.060
Sardine, canned	06.3	26.8	1.688	.140
Salmon	09.3	23.0	2.139	.053
Sablefish	10.0	22.9	2.290	.040
Mackerel, Atlantic	13.0	19.0	2.470	.065
Herring	15.0	18.4	2.760	.085
Dogfish shark	14.1	24.5	3.455	.039

[a]Data derived from the National Marine Fisheries Service and the scientific literature.

[b]Total percentages of 18:3w3, 20:5w3, 22:5w3, 22:6w3.

[c]Percent oil in flesh × percent omega-3 fatty acids in oil.

[d]Cholesterol percentages represent total cholesterol values. Note: The levels presented here are average figures. These levels may vary widely due to seasonality, fish diet, age, size, and the processing methods employed for the various product forms in which these fish species are sold to the public. Therefore, these figures should not be considered absolute.

Source: Barton and Emerson, 1986.

The author believes that physicians should recommend an increase in fish intake, so that fish is eaten at least twice weekly. Although all fish and shellfish contain omega-3 fatty acids, the amount contained in a single serving of one species can vary significantly from that contained in a single serving of another, owing to differences in their total oil content (Table 9). Generally speaking, a single serving of "lean" fish—those of low oil content—provides a lesser amount of omega-3 fatty acids than does a single serving of "oily" fish.

There is as yet no clear-cut evidence that indicates the optimal dose of omega-3 for either prophylactic or therapeutic use. The daily doses used in various studies have ranged from 0.54 g (Rice, 1983) to 4 g (Bradlow, 1986) and up to 12 g of omega-3 fatty acids per day in patients with hypertriglyceridemia (Phillipson et al., 1985). It appears as if the lowest daily dose of EPA that lowers blood pressure is 1.8 g EPA (Mortensen et al., 1983).

Supplements can be used by those who do not like fish and cannot obtain sufficient levels of omega-3 from their diets. An ideal supplement would contain high levels of EPA and DHA, with little or no cholesterol, vitamin A, or vitamin D. Vitamin E should be added as an antioxidant and preservative. Products are available which meet most of these requirements (Bradlow, 1986).

ACKNOWLEDGMENT

This work was supported by the Howard Heinz Endowment.

REFERENCES

Adam O, Wolfram G, Reiter S, Zollner N. Wirkung der Linol- und Linolensäure auf die Prostaglandinbildung und die Nierenfunktion biem Menschen. Fette, Seifen, Anstrichmittel 1984;86:180-191.

Aeberhard EE, Corbo L, Menkes JH. Polyenoic acid metabolism in cultured human skin fibroblasts. Lipids 1978;13:758-767.

Anderson RE. Lipids of ocular tissues. IV. A comparison of the phospholipids from the retina of six mammalian species. Exp Eye Res 1970;10:339.

Barton BM, Emerson JA. Seafood in your diet—a choice of recipes. In: Simopoulos AP, Kifer RR, Martin RE, eds. Health effects of polyunsaturated fatty acids in seafoods. Orlando, FL: Academic Press, 1986:403-430.

Benolken RM, Anderson RE, Wheeler TE. Membrane fatty acids associated with the electrical response in visual excitation. Science 1973;182:1253-1254.

Berry EM, Hirsch J. Does dietary linolenic acid influence blood pressure? Am J Clin Nutr 1986;44:336-340.

Bjerve KS. Letter to the editor. Am J Clin Nutr 1987;46:375-376.

Bjerve KS, Mostad IL, Thoresen L. Alpha-linolenic acid deficiency in patients on long-term gastric-tube feeding: estimation of linolenic acid and long-chain unsaturated n-3 fatty acid requirement in man. Am J Clin Nutr 1987;45:66-77.

Boudreau M, Chanmugam P, Hwang DH. Abstract 4966. Fed Proc 1987;46(4):1169.

Bradlow BA. Thrombosis and omega-3 fatty acids: epidemiological and clinical aspects. In: Simopoulos AP, Kifer RR, Martin RE, eds. Health effects of polyunsaturated fatty acids in seafoods. Orlando, FL: Academic Press, 1986:111-133.

Budowski P, Crawford MA. Alpha-linolenic acid as a regulator of the metabolism of arachidonic acid: dietary implications of the ratio, n-6, n-3 fatty acids. Proc Nutr Soc 1985;44:221-229.

Budowski P, Trostler N, Lupo M, Vaisman N, Eldor A. Effect of linseed oil ingestion on plasma fatty acid composition and platelet aggregability in healthy volunteers. Nutr Res 1984; 4:343-346.

Burr GO, Burr MM. A new deficiency disease produced by the rigid exclusion of fat from the diet. J Biol Chem 1929;82:345-367.

Burr GO, Burr MM. On the nature and role of fatty acids essential in nutrition. J Biol Chem 1930;86:587-621.

Carlson SE, Rhodes PG, Ferguson MG. Docosahexaenoic acid status of preterm infants at birth and following feeding with human milk or formula. Am J Clin Nutr 1986;44:798-804.

Cheek DB. In: Cheek DB, ed. Fetal and postnatal cellular growth: hormones and nutrition. New York, Wiley, 1975:3-22.

Clandinin MT, Chappell JE. Leong S, Heim T, Swyer PR, Chance GW. Intrauterine fatty acid accretion rates in human brain: implications for fatty acid requirements. Early Hum Dev 1980;4:121-129.

Clandinin MT, Chappell JE, Heim T, Swyer PR, Chance GW. Fatty acid accretion in fetal and neonatal liver: implications for fatty acid requirements. Early Hum Dev 1981a;5:1-6.

Clandinin MT, Chappell JE, Heim T, Swyer PR, Chance GW. Fatty acid utilization in perinatal de novo synthesis of tissues. Early Hum Dev 1981b;5:355-366.

Crawford MA. Fatty-acid ratios in free-living and domestic animals. Lancet 1968;1:1329-1333.

Crawford MA, Sinclair AJ. Nutritional influences in the evolution of the mammalian brain. In: Elliott K, and Knight J, eds. Lipids, malnutrition and the developing brain. Amsterdam: Associated Scientific Publishers, 1972;267-292.

Crawford MA, Gale MM, Woodford MH. Linoleic acid and linolenic acid elongation products in muscle tissue of Syncerus caffer and other ruminant species. Biochem J 1969;115:25-27.

Crawford MA, Sinclair AJ, Msuya PM, Munhambo A. Structural lipids and their polyenoic constituents in human milk. In: Galli C, Jacini G, Pecile A, eds. Dietary lipids and postnatal development. New York: Raven Press, 1973:41.

Crawford MA, Hassam AG, Williams G. Essential fatty acids and fetal brain growth. Lancet 1976 2:452-453.

Crawford MA, Hassam AG, Stevens PA. Essential fatty acid requirements in pregnancy and lactation with special reference to brain development. Prog Lipid Res 1981;20:31-40.

de Gomez Dumm INT, Brenner RR. Oxidative desaturation of alpha-linolenic, linoleic, and stearic acids by human liver microsomes. Lipids 1975;10:315-317.

Deuel HJ Jr. The lipids. Vol. 1. New York: Interscience, 1951:18.

Fiennes RNTW, Sinclair AJ, Crawford MA. Essential fatty acid studies in primates, linolenic acid requirements of capuchins. J Med Prim 1973;2:155-169.

Friedman Z, Frolich J. Essential fatty acids and the major urinary metabolites of the E prostaglandins in thriving neonates and in infants receiving parenteral fat emulsions. Pediatr Res 1979;13:932-936.

Galli C, Trzeciak HI, Paoletti R. Effects of dietary fatty acids on the fatty acid composition of brain ethanolamine phosphoglyceride. Reciprocal replacement of n-6 and n-3 polyunsaturated fatty acids. Biochim Biophys Acta 1971a;248:449-454.

Galli C, White HB Jr, Paoletti R. Lipid alterations and their reversion in the central nervous system of growing rats deficient in essential fatty acids. Lipids 1971b;6:378-387.

Galli C, Agradi E, Paoletti R. The (n-6) pentaene: (n-3) hexane fatty acid ratio as an index of linolenic acid deficiency. Biochim Biophys Acta 1974;369:142-145.

Hague TA, Christoffersen BO. Effect of dietary fats on arachidonic acid and eicosapentaenoic acid biosynthesis and conversion to C_{22} fatty acids in isolated liver cells. Biochim Biophys Acta 1984;796:205-217.

Hague TA, Christoffersen BO. Evidence for peroxisomal retroconversion of adrenic acid (22:4n6) and docosahexaenoic acid (22:6n3) in isolated liver cells. Biochim Biophys Acta 1986;875:165-173.

Hansen AE, Haggard M, Boelsche A, Adam D, Wiese H. Essential fatty acid in infant nutrition. III. Clinical manifestations of linoleic acid deficiency. J Nutr 1958;66:565-576.

Hansen HS. The essential nature of linoleic acid in mammals. Trends Biochem Sci 1986;11:263-265.

Harris WS, Connor WE, Lindsey S. Will dietary omega-3 fatty acids change the composition of human milk? Am J Clin Nutr 1984;40:780-785.

Hilditch TP, Williams PN. The chemical constitution of natural fats. 4th ed. London: Chapman and Hall, 1964.

Hirsch J, Farquhar JW, Ahrens EH Jr, Peterson ML, Stoffel W. Studies of adipose tissue in man: a micro-technique for sampling and analysis. Am J Clin Nutr 1960;8:499-511.

Holman RT. The ratio of trienoic:tetraenoic acids in tissue lipids as a measure of essential fatty acid requirement. J Nutr 1960;70:405-410.

Holman RT. Progress in the chemistry of fats and other lipids. Vol. IX. New York: Pergammon Press, 1970:275-348.

Holman RT, Johnson SB, Hatch TF. A case of human linolenic acid deficiency involving neurological abnormalities. Am J Clin Nutr 1982;35:617-623.

Holt LE, Tidwell HC, Kirk CM, Cross DM, Neale S. Studies in fat metabolism: fat absorption in normal infants. J Pediatr 1935;6:427-480.

Honigmann G, Schimke E, Beitz J, Mest HJ, Schliack V. Influence of a diet rich in linolenic acid on lipids, thrombocyte aggregation and prostaglandins in type I (insulin-dependent) diabetes. Diabetologia 1982;23:175.

Hyman BT, Spector AA. Accumulation of n-3 polyunsaturated fatty acids by cultured human Y79 retinoblastoma cells. J Neurochem 1981;37:60-69.

Innis SM. Effect of total parenteral nutrition with linoleic acid-rich emulsions on tissue w6 and w3 fatty acids in the rat. Lipids 1986;21:132-138.

Johnston PV, Fritsche KL. Linolenate metabolism. Nutr Rev 1986;44;315-316.

Kamada T, Yamashita T, Baba Y, et al. Dietary sardine oil increases erythrocyte membrane fluidity in diabetic patients. Diabetes 1986;35:604-611.

King ME, Spector AA. Effect of specific fatty acyl enrichments on membrane physical properties detected with a spin label probe. J Biol Chem 1978;253:6493-6501.

Koletzko B. Letter to the editor. Am J Clin Nutr 1987;46:374.

Lamptey MS, Walker BL. A possible essential role for dietary linolenic acid in the development of the young rat. J Nutr 1976;106:86-93.

Ledger HP. Body composition as a basis for a comparative study of some East African mammals. Symp Zool Soc London 1968;21:289-310.

Liu C-CF, Carlson SE, Rhodes PG, Rao VS, Meydrech EF. Increase in plasma phospholipid docosahexaenoic and eicosapentaenoic acids as a reflection of their intake and mode of administration. Pediatr Res 1987;22:292-296.

Martinez M, Ballabriga A. Effects of parenteral nutrition with high doses of linoleate on the developing human liver and brain. Lipids 1987;22:133-138.

Martinez M, Ballabriga A. A chemical study on the development of the human forebrain and cerebellum during the brain "growth spurt" period. I. Gangliosides and plasmalogens. Brain Res 1978;159:351-362.

Martinez M, Conde C, Ballabriga A. Some chemical aspects of human brain development. II. Phosphaglyceride fatty acids. Pediatr Res 1974;8:93-102.

Mest H-J, Beitz J, Heinroth I, Block H-U, Forster W. The influence of linseed oil diet on fatty acid pattern in phospholipids and thromboxane formation in platelets in man. Klin Wochenschr. 1983;61:187-191.

Mortensen JZ, Schmidt EB, Nielsen AH, et al. The effect of n-6 and n-3 polyunsaturated fatty acids on homeostasis, blood lipids and blood pressure. Thromb Haemost 1983;50:543-546.

Needleman P, Raz A, Minkes MS, Ferrendeli JA, Sprecher H. Triene prostaglandins: prostacyclin and thromboxane biosynthesis and unique biological properties. Proc Natl Acad Sci USA 1979;76:944-948.

Neuringer M, Connor WE, Petten CV, Barstad L. Dietary omega-3 fatty acid deficiency and visual loss in infant rhesus monkeys. J Clin Invest 1984;73:272-276.

Neuringer M, Connor WE, Lin DS, Barstad L, Luck S. Biochemical and functional effects of prenatal and postnatal w-3 fatty acid deficiency on retina and brain in rhesus monkeys. Proc Natl Acad Sci USA 1986;83:4021-4025.

O'Brien JS, Sampson EL. Fatty acid and aldehyde composition of the major brain lipids in normal gray matter, white matter and myelin. J Lipid Res 1965;6:545-551.

Olsen SF, Hansen HS, Jensen B et al. Duration of pregnancy and intake of marine fat in two populations, one with low and one with high consumption of marine fat. In: Lands WEM, ed. Proceedings of the AOCS short course on polyunsaturated fatty acids and eicosanoids. Champaign, Illinois: American Oil Chemists Society, 1987: 268-269.

Olsen SF, Joensen HD. High liveborn birth weights in the Faroes: a comparison between birth weights in the Faroes and in Denmark. J Epidemiol Comm Health 1985;39:27-32.

Olsen SF, Hansen HS, Sorensen TIA, Jensen B, Secher NJ, Sommer S, Knudsen LB. Intake of marine fat, rich in (n-3)-polyunsaturated fatty acids, may increase birthweight by prolonging gestation. Lancet 1986;2:367-369.

Paoletti R, Galli C. Effects of essential fatty acid deficiency on the central nervous system in the growing rat. In: Elliott K, Knight J, eds. Lipids, malnutrition and the developing brain. Amsterdam: Associated Scientific Publishers, 1972: 121-140.

Phillipson BE, Rothrock DW, Connor WE et al. Reduction of plasma lipid, lipoproteins and apoproteins by dietary fish oils in patients with hypertriglyceridemia. N Engl J Med 1985;312: 1210-1216.

Poulos A, Darin-Bennett A, White IG. The phospholipid bound fatty acids and aldehydes of mammalian spermatozoa. Comp Biochem Physiol 1975;46B:541.

Renaud S, Nordoy A. Small is beautiful: alpha-linolenic acid and eicosapentaenoic acid in man. Lancet 1983;1:1169.

Renaud S, Dumont E, Godsey F, et al. Dietary fats and platelet function in French and Scottish farmers. Nutr Metab 1980; 24:90-104.

Renaud S, Godsey F, Dumont E, Thevenon C, Ortchanian E, Martin J. Influence of long-term diet modification on platelet function and composition in Moselle farmers. Am J Clin Nutr 1986;43:136-150.

Rice DR. The effects of low doses of Max EPA for long periods. Br J Clin Pract 1983;81(Suppl):85-95.

Rotstein NP, Ilincheta de Boschero MG, Giusto NM, Alveldano MI. Effects of aging on the composition and metabolism of docosahexaenoate-containing lipids of retina. Lipids 1987; 22:253-260.

Salem N Jr, Kim HY, Yergey JA. Docosahexaenoic acid: membrane function and metabolism. In: Simopoulos AP, Kifer RR, Martin RE, eds. Health effects of polyunsaturated fatty acids in seafoods. Orlando, FL: Academic Press, 1986:263-317.

Sanders TAB, Naismith DJ. Long-chain polyunsaturated fatty acids in the erythrocyte lipids of breast-fed and bottle-fed infants. Proc Nutr Soc 1976;64A.

Sanders TAB, Younger KM. The effect of dietary supplements of omega-3 polyunsaturated fatty acids on the fatty acid composition of platelets and plasma choline phosphoglycerides. Br J Nutr 1981;45:613-616.

Sanders TAB, Ellis FR, Dickerson JWT. Studies in vegans: the fatty acid composition of plasma choline phosphoglycerides, erythrocytes, adipose tissue and breast milk, and some indicators of susceptibility to ischemic heart disease in vegans and normal controls. Am J Clin Nutr 1978;31:805-813.

Simopoulos AP, Grave GD. Infant-Feeding Task Force Report. Section III. Factors associated with the choice and duration of infant-feeding practice. Pediatrics 1984;74:603-614.

Simopoulos AP, Salem N Jr. Purslane: a terrestrial source of omega-3 fatty acids. N Engl J Med 1986;315:833.

Simopoulos AP, Kifer RR, Martin RE, eds. Health effects of poly-unsaturated fatty acids in seafoods. Orlando FL: Academic Press, 1986.

Storlien LH, Kraegen EW, Chisholm DJ, Ford GL, Bruce DG, Pascoe WS. Fish oil prevents insulin resistance induced by high-fat feeding in rats. Science 1987;237:885-888.

Svennerholm L. Distribution and fatty acid composition of phos-phoglycerides in normal human brain. J Lipid Res 1968; 9:570-579.

Von Groer F. Zur frage der praktischen bedeutung des nahrwert-begriffes nebt einigen menschlichen sauglings. Biochem Z 1919;97:311-329.

Walker BL. Maternal diet and brain fatty acids in young rats. Lipids 1967;2:497-500.

Weber PC, Fischer S, Von Schacky C, Lorenz R, Strasser T. Diet-ary omega-3 polyunsaturated fatty acids and eicosanoid for-mation in man. In: Simopoulos AP, Kifer RR, Martin RE, eds. Health effects of polyunsaturated fatty acids in sea-foods. Orlando, FL: Academic Press, 1986:49-60.

Wheeler TG, Benolken RM, Anderson RE. Visual membranes: specificity of fatty acid precursors for the electrical response to illumination. Science 1975;188:1312-1314.

Witting LA. The interrelationship of polyunsaturated fatty acids and antioxidants in vivo. Prog Chem Fats 1970;9:517-553.

Witting LA, Harvey CC, Century B, Horwitt MK. Dietary altera-tions of fatty acids of erythrocytes and mitochondria of brain and liver. J Lipid Res 1961;2:412-418.

Wo CKW, Draper HH. Vitamin E status of Alaskan Eskimos. Am J Clin Nutr 1975;28:808-813.

Zimmerman T, Winkler L, Moller U, Schubert H, Goetze E. Syn-thesis of arachidonic acid in the human placenta in vitro. Biol Neonate 1979;35:209-212.

Part II: Sources of Dietary and Pharmacological Omega-3 Fatty Acids

7
Sources of Omega-3 Fatty Acids in Human Diets

John E. Kinsella
Institute of Food Science, Cornell University
Ithaca, New York

INTRODUCTION

The burgeoning information from epidemiological and clinical studies concerning the apparent beneficial effects of n-3 polyunsaturated fatty acids (n-3 PUFA) underscores the limited understanding of the discrete functions of and interactions between dietary unsaturated fatty acids as they affect numerous physiological functions. Notwithstanding the recent developments concerning the effects of PUFA (Lands, 1986; Simopoulos et al., 1986), there is still a need for research to elucidate the biochemistry, enzymology, and regulation of PUFA metabolism and the mechanisms of eicosanoid action, because an understanding of these phenomena is necessary to discuss intelligently the human requirements for PUFA.

The PUFA of interest here are those of the n-6 and n-3 families (Fig. 1), which use common enzymatic pathways for elonga-

Families of Dietary Polyunsaturated Fatty Acids (PUFA)

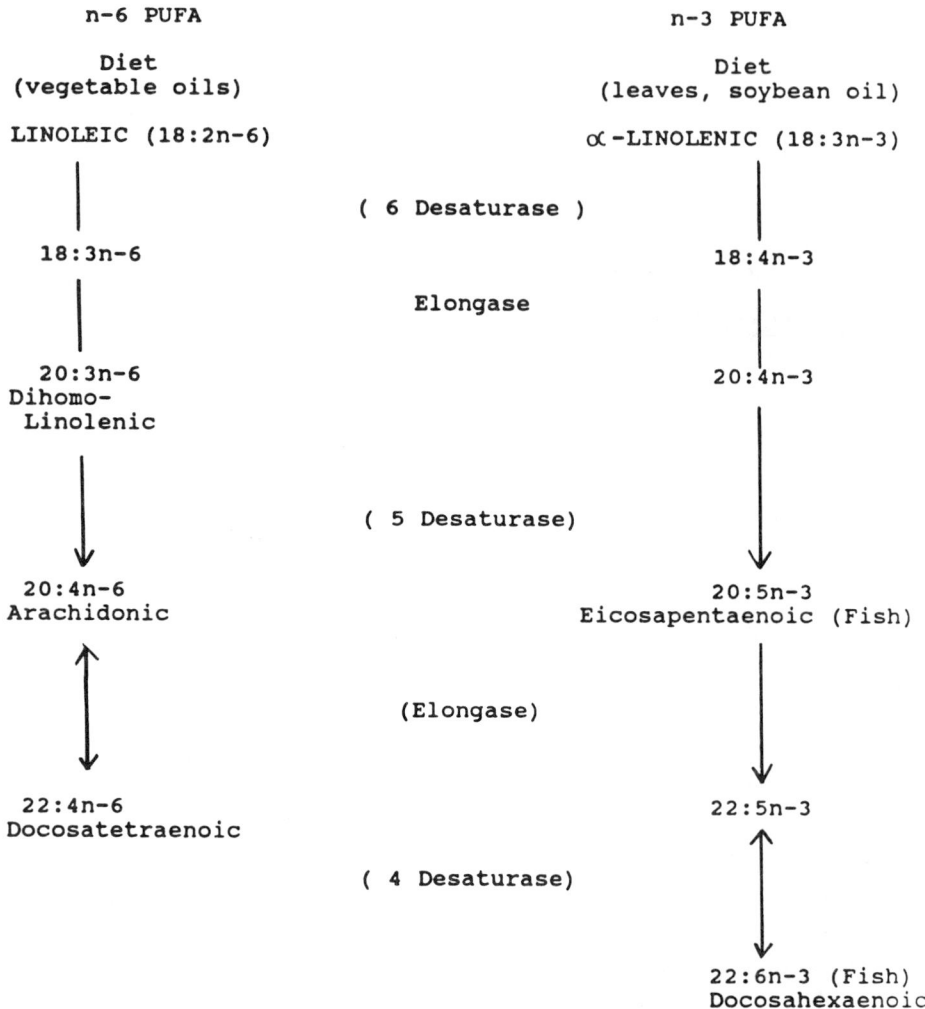

Figure 1   The elongation and desaturation of the two major families of dietary unsaturated fatty acids in foods. Linoleic acid (18: 2n-6) is abundant in vegetable oils (soybean, corn, safflower); linolenic acid 18:3n-3 occurs in low concentrations in leafy plant tissues, canola, and soybean oil. These fatty acids are sequentially desaturated and elongated by desaturases and elongase enzymes present in liver and tissues. Eicosapentaenoic acids (EPA, 20:5n -3) and docosahexaenoic acid (DHA, 22:6n-3), abundant in fish oil, occur in low concentrations in tissues from persons on normal diet, but these are increased in subjects consuming seafood and marine oils.

tion and desaturation (Sprecher, 1986). Early work on essential fatty acids established that the minimum requirement for growth and prevention of deficiency symptoms was approximately 1.5 energy percent (en%) linoleic acid 18:2n-6, corresponding to approximately 3 g/day. Though the PUFA of the n-3 family exert some ameliorating effects on deficiency symptoms, they cannot substitute for n-6 PUFA (Holman, 1986). It was speculated that the PUFA of the n-6 family were essential for membrane integrity, and recently their role as integral components of skin acyl-ceramides (which control epidermal water permeation) was reported (Wertz, 1986). However, the discovery and elucidation of the synthesis and diverse metabolic effects of eicosanoids (Gerrard, 1985; Bailey, 1986; Lands, 1986) dramatically clarified the major essential functions of n-6 dietary PUFA (Fig. 2). The biological effects of these eicosanoids in modulating numerous physiological functions (Table 1) have cogently underscored the critical role of dietary n-6 PUFA in human health (Lands, 1986). Nevertheless, the optimum intake of dietary n-6 PUFA for eicosanoid homeostasis has not been established. Presumably, this may vary with gender, age, physiological state, disease, and other dietary factors.

LINOLENIC ACID

Fatty acids of the n-3 family are normal components of foods, especially leafy foods and seafoods. Linolenic acid occurs in the triglycerides of some plant oils, and green leaves/vegetables and is readily available following digestion (Zollner, 1986). Dietary n-3 PUFA, especially 18:3n-3 from plants, is metabolized preponderantly to 22:6n-3 (DHA) by the same desaturases and elongases that transform 18:2n-6 to 20:4n-6 (AA) (Sprecher, 1986) (Fig. 1). Unlike 20:4n-6, DHA is normally incorporated selectively into particular tissues in the body, i.e., neural cells and synapse membranes, outer rod segments of the eye, and sperm tissue (Tinoco, 1982). Though its specific function(s) have not been determined, DHA may somehow be involved in mechanisms related to nerve

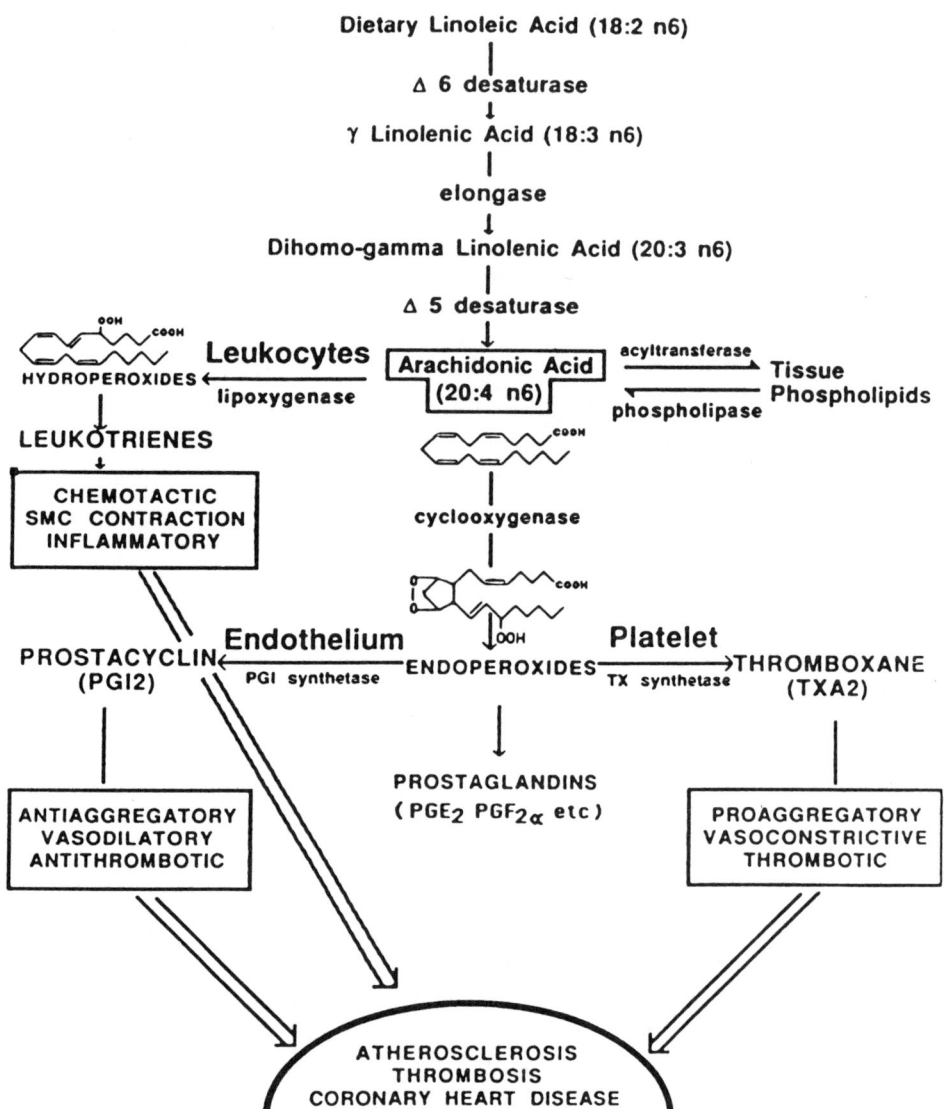

transmission, vision (visual acuity), and sperm motility (Tinoco, 1982; Dyerberg, 1986; Bjerve et al., 1987a; Zollner, 1986).

A human requirement for n-3 PUFA has not been estblished though evidence for deficiency in humans and primates has been reported (Zollner, 1986; Tinoco, 1982). It appears that n-3 PUFA as linolenic 18:3n-3 or long-chain n-3 PUFA (EPA, DHA) is re-

---

Figure 2 The conversion of dietary linoleic acid to arachidonic acid and thence to eicosanoids. Lipoxygenase generates hydroperoxides, which are converted to leukotriens and hydroxy fatty acids. These are very important mediators of leukocyte (monocyte, macrophage, neutrophil) functions and may play a role in atherogenesis. The leukotriene LTB_4 is a potent chemoattractant for neutrophils and induces aggregation, oxidative metabolism, and inflammation. In 18:2n6 deficiency LTB_4 formation is reduced and neutrophil activation may be impaired or in EFA excess it may be enhanced. The slow-reacting substances of anaphylaxis, i.e., leukotrienes LTC_4, D_4, and E_4 derived from AA, are potent bronchioconstrictive agents both in vivo and in vitro; they induce contraction of bronchial and vascular smooth muscle, induce tracheal edema, and stimulate mucus hypersecretion. These peptidoleukotrienes act as mediators of anaphylactic reactions and contribute to the pathophysiology of allergic asthma. Since these leukotrienes are generated by 5-lipoxygenase, inhibitors of this lipoxygenase are of interest. The n-3 PUFA may be effective in this regard. Cyclooxygenase generate endoperoxides which are converted to prostanoids with differing functions according to tissue; e.g., thromboxane produced in platelets is thrombotic, whereas prostacyclin produced by endothelial cells counteracts these effects. Other prostaglandins with various functions are produced in other tissues. An imbalance or excess may result in pathological states. Dietary n-3 polyunsaturated fatty acids may modulate eicosanoid production by reducing arachidonic acid synthesis via inhibition of 6-desaturase by inhibition of cyclooxygenase and lipoxygenase. This can reduce pathophysiologies, relieve PGE_2-induced immunosuppressive effects, and reduce inflammation, endotoxic shock, etc. (see text for references).

Table 1 Some Biological Functions of Prostanoids and Leukotrienes

Organ system	Effects	Active species
Prostanoids		
Blood vessels	Vasodilation	$PGI_2 > PGI_3 > PGE_1$
	Vasoconstriction	TXA_2
Platelets	Adhesion, aggregation	TXA_2
	Antiaggregatory	$PGI_2 > PGI_3 > PGE$
Lung	Bronchiole constriction	PGF_2, TXA_2, PGD_2
	Bronchiole dilation	PGE_2, PGI_2
Kidney	Glomerular filtration rate	TXA_2, PGE_2, PGE_2
	Renin secretion	PGI_2, PGF_2
	Natriuresis	PGE_2, PGI_2
	Diuresis	PGE_2
Stomach	Acid secretion	PGE_2, PGE_1
Small intestine	Peristalsis	PGE_2, PGF_2
Pancreas	Amylase secretion	PGI_2, PGI_2
	Insulin secretion	PGE_2
Hypophysis	Secretion (growth hormone, adreno-corticotropic hormone)	PGE_2
Tissue	Pain	PGE_2
	Cytoprotection	PGI_2, dimethyl PGE_2
Leukotrienes		
Bronchioles	Constriction	LTC_4, LTD_4
Ileum	Constriction	LTC_4, LTD_4
Vascular	Constriction	LTC_4, LTD_4
	Permeability	LTC_4, LTD_4
Pancreas	Insulin secretion	LTB_4, HETE
Neutrophils	Adhesion	LTB_4
	Chemotaxis/kinesis	LTB_4, HETE
	Lysozyme secretion	LTB_4, HETE
Monocytes	Chemotaxis/kinesis	LTB_4, HETE (5,9,11)
Basophils	Histamine secretion	LTB_4, HETEs

PG = prostaglandin; PGI_2 = prostacyclin; TXA = thromboxane; LT = leukotriene; HETE = hydroxyeicosatetraenoic acid.

quired for nerve tissue and brain development (learning), for visual acuity, and for sperm function. In addition, it may function in modulating eicosanoid production. Insofar as n-3 PUFA cannot be synthesized in mammalian tissue, it may be considered an essential dietary component. However, the precise quantitative requirements for n-3 PUFA have not been established. Presumably, these are higher in the developing fetus, the nursing mother, sexually active males, and older subjects where desaturase activity is low. Teleologically, it is generally suggested that n-3 PUFA is needed for optimum development of brain and eye, particularly during the first 12 months of human development (Budowski and Crawford, 1985).

Evidence of deficiencies of n-3 PUFA is sparse (Zollner, 1986). Holman (1982) reported that dietary linolenic acid relieved neurological symptoms (numbness, weakness, periodic inability to walk, blurring of vision) in a 6-year-old girl on parenteral nutrition. Recently, Bjerve et al. (1987b) reported on four adults suffering from a deficiency of 18:3n-3. Patients on a parenteral protein-rich diet, deficient in 18:3n-3, developed scaly dermatitis on the shoulders, with general skin atrophy and excoriations. Supplementation with ethyl linolenic corrected this and greatly increased the EPA and DHA levels in blood cell lipids. Supplementation of 100 mg of ethyl 18:3n-3 for 14 days did not cause a significant change in 18:3 or 20:5n-3 in erythrocytes, but 22:5n-3 and 22:6n-3 increased threefold. Coincidentally AA levels increased and the scaly dermatitis nearly disappeared. The data indicate that 18:3n-3 can be converted relatively rapidly to DHA in these human subjects on low-fat diets. These patients also responded to cod liver oil containing preformed DHA. Neuringer and Connor (1986) reported that a deficiency of 18:3n-3 resulted in visual impairment in primates and humans.

Based on their observations, Holman and Johnson (1982) and Bjerve et al. (1987a) suggested an 18:3n-3 requirement of approximately 20 mg/kg/day. This may greatly depend on stage of development, age, gender, physiology and dietary n-6 PUFA intake. The longer-chain n-3 PUFAs, i.e., EPA and DHA, are probably more effective than 18:3n-3. Thus, an average person may require 3 g n-3 PUFA, which could be provided by 40 g of soybean oil, 35 g of canola oil, 1 kg of leafy vegetables, 120 g of salmon with 10% fat, 800 g of sole, 15 g of maxEPA, or 150 g of butterfat. Zollner (1986) suggested that 0.5 en% calories from 18:3n-3 is perhaps a high estimate and humans can survive with much less. However, the amounts required (perhaps as a precursor of DHA) are greatly affected by the level of 18:2n-6 in the diet (which inhibits conversion to 22:6n-3). Furthermore, the minimum may be sufficient to avoid overt symptoms of deficiency, such as impaired vision, but higher levels may be desirable in diets containing large amounts of 18:2n-6 to modulate eicosanoid synthesis.

Dietary linolenic acid is incorporated into phospholipids (PL) and cholesterol esters (CE) of plasma lipids in a dose-dependent manner. Usually incorporation occurs at the expense of oleic acid with limited effects on 18:2n-6 or AA. The rate and extent of incorporation of linolenic acid is less when 18:2 is fed in the diet. Much less EPA accumulates in plasma lipids after feeding 18:3n-3 than upon feeding EPA itself. This indicates that 18:3n-3 is only slowly converted to EPA. Dietary 18:3n-3 reduces plasma eicosanoids (Quadt and TenHoor, 1982; Jacotot et al., 1986).

FACTORS AFFECTING DOSAGE OF n-3 PUFA

No systematic study to determine optimum n-3 intake in humans for either prophylactic or therapeutic purposes has been reported, and relatively few well-designed or -controlled clinical trials have been conducted (Herold and Kinsella, 1986). Therefore, only tentative suggestions can be made, based on epidemiological and scattered clinical trials which have recently been summarized (Kinsella, 1987a).

In the context of this discussion, relevant factors that govern the metabolic efficacy of n-3 PUFA (i.e., fat content and fatty acid composition of the diet), the n-3 species used, and the particular physiological parameter being studied must be assessed (Fig. 3). Tissue antioxidant status (dietary tocopherol, vitamin C, phenolics, flavanoids, selenium, glutathione, peroxidase, etc.)

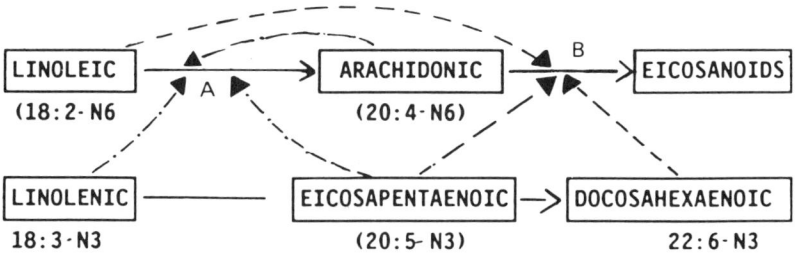

Figure 3 Loci of inhibition of tissue eicosanoid biosynthesis by dietary polyunsaturated fatty acids. (A) 6-desaturase; (B) cyclooxygenase and lipoxygenase.

may greatly affect the metabolic efficacy of n-3 PUFA on eicosanoid synthesis. Nonsteroidal antiinflammatory agents such as aspirin can also affect actions of n-3 PUFA. These variables need to be defined and are briefly discussed below (Table 2). In animal trials, increasing fat content of diets tend to suppress the efficacy of dietary n-3 PUFA in inhibiting eicosanoid synthesis by microphages (German et al., 1988).

Because dietary n-3 PUFA affect different parameters and pathophysiological symptoms via different mechanisms, there may be an optimum dietary intake for each of these. Dietary n-3 PUFA may act directly, e.g., suppression of hepatic lipid and lipo-

Table 2 Some Factors Affecting Efficacy of Dietary n-3 PUFA

1. Total fat consumption
2. Composition of dietary fat (i.e., n6:n3 ratio)
3. Type of n-3 polyunsaturated fatty acid linolenic vs. eicosapentaenoic vs. docosahexaenoic acid
4. Antioxidant status (peroxide tone)
        Tocopherol, phenolics, flavanoids
        Selenium glutathione peroxidase
5. Nonsteroidal antiinflammatory agents
        Aspirin; indomethacin

Table 3 Possible Role or Mode of Action of n-3 Polyunsaturated
Fatty Acids on Functions Mediated by n-6 Polyunstaturated Fatty
Acids

Impair uptake of n-6 polyunsaturated fatty acids (PUFA)
Inhibit desaturases, especially Δ-6-desaturase
Compete with n-6 PUFA for acyltransferases
Displace arachidonic acid from specific PL pools
Dilute pools of free arachidonic acid (AA)
Competitively inhibit cyclooxygenase and lipoxygenase
Form eicosanoid analogs with less activity or competitively bind to
    eicosanoid sites
Alter membrane properties and associated enzyme and receptor
    functions

---

protein synthesis (Saynor et al., 1986; Harris, 1989; Sanders
et al., 1985; Wong and Nestel, 1987). However, it appears that
the effects of dietary n-3 PUFA are exerted via their action on
eicosanoid-related phenomena (Table 3). This reflects competition of n-3 PUFA with the metabolism of 18:2n-6 to 20:4-n-6,
thereby limiting the substrate for eicosanoid synthesis, via competitive inhibition of the enzymes cyclooxygenase and lipoxygenase, which synthesize the bioactive prostanoids, leukotrienes,
and lipoxins, and perhaps via n-3 PUFA conversion to less active
eicosanoid analogs.

In this regard, the concentration of n-6 PUFA in the diet
greatly affects the efficacy of n-3 PUFA, particularly dietary 18:
3n-3 (Hwang et al., 1988), the potency of which depends significantly on its conversion to 20:5n-3 and 22:6n-3. Thus, 18:2n-6
effectively competes for the initial rate-limiting Δ5 desaturase step
and minimizes the conversion of 18:3 to 20:5n-3 and 22:6n-3,
respectively. Because of this, the effective dose of n-3 PUFA has
to be increased as the quantity of dietary 18:2 is increased and
the dose of n-3 PUFA can be decreased when intake of n-6 PUFA
is reduced. Significantly, Nikkari (1986) showed that in Finnish
subjects safflower oil (30 ml/day) caused an increase in plasma
18:2n-6 which was accompanied by a disproportionately large de-

crease in the n-3 PUFA of all lipid fractions. The mean 18:2n-6-to-18:3n-3 ratio increased from 67 to 75 to 181 and 200, in plasma CE and PL, respectively, after 6 weeks. Thus, high dietary linoleate, by competing for desaturases, elongases, and acyltransferases, may result in a relative depletion of n-3 PUFA.

The effectiveness of the long-chain n-3 PUFAs, especially EPA and DHA, reflects their potency as competitive inhibitors of cyclooxygenase (Ki 2 μM) and lipoxygenase (Ki 2-4 μM) (Lands et al., 1973). Therefore, their efficacy is enhanced when the tissue concentrations of 18:2n-6 and 20:4n-6 are low, i.e., when dietary 18:2n-6 is restricted.

Because the activity of the oxygenases is dependent on a relatively high (10^{-8} M) acyl hydroperoxide tone (Lands and Kulmacz, 1986) and because arachidonyl hydroperoxide is an order of magnitude more active than the corresponding hydroperoxides of EPA and DHA, the endogenous peroxide tone is another mechanism by which the concentration of n-6 PUFA affects the effectiveness of n-3 PUFA in down-regulating eicosanoid synthesis in tissues.

The n-3 PUFA may also function by altering the physical properties of membranes, thereby modifying the activities of membrane-associated enzymes and receptors, which in turn can affect specific physiological functions, e.g., calcium ATPase, 5'nucleotidase, and andrenergic receptors (Flier et al., 1985; Salem, 1986). Such effects may reflect the capacity of n-3 PUFA to displace n-6 PUFA from membrane lipids, e.g., the selective acylation of DHA into cardiac sacroplasmic reticulum (Swanson et al., 1987). Thus, in terms of eicosanoid-mediated functions, the effective dosage of dietary n-3 PUFA is principally influenced by the concomitant intake of n-6 PUFA, especially 18:2n-6. This is relevant in assessing human dietary needs for and sources of n-3 PUFA for the amelioration of eicosanoid-related physiopathologies.

Generally, in human clinical trials very high doses of n-3 PUFA (from fish, fish oils) have been employed. These have ranged from 5 to 50 g of fish oil per day (i.e., approximately 1-10 g n-3 PUFA per day) and generally have caused significant

effects on the various (mostly related to cardiovascular) parameters studied (Kinsella, 1987b). However, subjects have varied
from healthy to ill; they have differed in age; and duration of
intervention has been short and in very few studies have other
dietary factors been monitored, much less controlled. The studies
of Saynor et al. (1986), Sanders et al. (1985), von Schacky et al.
(1986), Knapp et al. (1986), Connor et al. (1969); Connor (1986);
Lee et al. (1985), and others (Herold and Kinsella, 1986) indicate
that doses greater than 3 g n-3 PUFA per day have measurable,
desirable effects on plasma lipids, proaggregatory eicosanoids, and
inflammatory and arthritic ailments.

   Saynor et al. (1986) conducted several trials (open and
double-blind) in which maxEPA was administered to patients with
myocardial infarction, hypertension, peripheral vascular disease,
and elevated plasma triglycerides. Fish oil was fed (10 ml or 1.8 g
n-3 PUFA) twice daily with normal food and compared with similar amounts of n-6 PUFA in capsules containing peppermint fla-
voring. Fish oil consumption caused marked decreases in plasma
triglycerides from 3.5 to 2 mmol/liter. The response was greater
in hypertriglyceridemic patients. A significant decrease in total
serum cholesterol and in very-low-density lipoprotein (VLDL) and
an increase in high-density lipoprotein was observed. Bleeding
time increased from 3.6 to 7 min and glyceryl trinitrate consumption in 12 subjects decreased from 25 to 2 tablets/week. These
effects were persistent with continued ingestion of fish oil. Similar results have been reported by Sanders et al. (1985) and Connor
(1986).

   Dietary EPA reduces VLDL synthesis (Iritani et al., 1980;
Daggy et al., 1987; Wong and Nestel, 1987). The n-3 PUFA may
also increase VLDL clearance. This may reflect a more favorable
ratio of PGI_1 :TXA in plasma, rather than any specific increase
in lipoprotein lipase per se. Saynor et al. (1986) concluded that
inclusion of n-3 PUFA in the normal diet may be useful in mini-
mizing coronary heart disease.

   In free-living Finnish populations, a positive correlation between the saturated fatty acids in platelets and adrenaline-induced
aggregation was observed. A negative relationship between the n-3

PUFA and aggregation was observed for both ADP and adrenaline, even at an average EPA level of 1.8%, in the presence of 8% AA and 20% 18:2n-6 in plasma phospholipids (Salo, 1986).

Generally, dietary n-3 PUFAs are effective when they displace AA from eicosanoid-specific phospholipid pools in the various tissues. Hence, monitoring the level of the n-3 PUFA in tissue PL pools, e.g., plasma, platelet, or monocyte phospholipids, may provide a good index of the effectiveness of dosage. However, this may be influenced by the relative concentration of AA; hence the ratio of AA to n-3 PUFA in PL of particular tissues may be a more reliable index of n-3 PUFA adequacy (Knapp et al., 1986; von Schacky et al., 1986). In this regard, the ratio in phosphatidylethanolamine (PE), the most sensitive PL class to AA replacement by n-3 PUFA, may be the phospholipid to monitor (Swanson et al., 1987, 1988).

Analyses of tissue PL of Eskimo or Japanese subjects who routinely consume seafood (and who from epidemiological studies have a low incidence of atherosclerosis, thrombosis, and heart disease) reveal extensive replacement of AA by n-3 PUFA, i.e., EPA and DHA (Dyerburg et al., 1975; Kagawa et al., 1982). Thus in Japanese subjects consuming approximately 100 and 250 g seafood per day, the AA:n-3 PUFA ratio in serum phospholipids was 1:1.5 and 1:2, respectively, compared to 30:1 in subjects in the United States consuming negligible quantities of seafood (Yamori et al., 1985). Knapp et al. (1986) showed that administration of 10 g EPA per day to healthy subjects reduced the AA:n-3 PUFA ratio from approximately 50:1 to 5:1 in serum phosphatidylethanolamine and from 13:1 to 1:1 in phosphatidylcholine after 2-3 weeks. von Schacky et al. (1985a,b) observed that consumption of increasing levels of cod liver oil by young men who consumed a normal diet (the lipid content and composition of which were unreported) caused a progressive decrease in plasma AA with a concurrent increase in n-3 PUFA in phospholipids and cholesterol esters.

These and other studies (Herold and Kinsella, 1986; Harris, 1989) have reported favorable changes in plasma lipids, especially triglycerides, reduction in proaggregatory thromboxane, reduction

in blood pressure, and in some cases relief from angina and pain
related to inflammation and arthritis (Saynor et al., 1986; Lands,
1987; Simopoulos et al., 1986; Leaf and Weber, 1988). Since
many of these studies lacked appropriate controls, their findings
cannot be considered definitive.

SPECIES OF n-3 PUFA

The species of n-3 fatty acids in the diet may also determine the
threshold for the appearance of a metabolic effect. Generally,
the elongated polyunsaturated n-3 acids, i.e., EPA and DHA, are
more potent and more immediate in their effects on plasma lipids
and eicosanoids than their normal dietary precursor linolenic
acid 18:3n-3. This is because 18:3n-3 has to be desaturated and
elongated to EPA and DHA mostly in liver, and the desaturase is
easily inhibited by dietary 18:2n-6 (Sprecher, 1986; Hwang et al.
1988). In this regard the desaturases in the liver may regulate
PUFA levels available to cardiovascular tissues and cells (especially platelets and macrophages) which lack desaturase. Hence,
for these tissues the preformed long-chain n-3 PUFA are superior
to dietary 18:3n-3 in displacing AA and inhibiting the oxygenases
involved in eicosanoid synthesis.

　　Nevertheless, the studies of Renaud (1987) and Nikkari
(1986) and trials with linseed oil (55% 18:3n-3) indicate that
dietary 18:3n-3, when ingested as part of the normal diet, can
increase tissue levels of n-3 PUFA and reduce AA and eicosanoids (Jacotot et al., 1986; Quadt and TenHoor, 1986; Zollner,
1986; Hwang et al., 1988). The work of Renaud (1987) indicates that long-term ingestion of 18:3n-3 results in a small, but significant increase in EPA and DHA levels in tissue phospholipids.
These apparently are effective in reducing platelet aggregation in
humans. When daily intake of 18:3n-3 was increased from 0.3 to
1.0 en%, a significant increase in platelet phospholipid n-3 PUFA
(from 0.3 to 0.5%) occurred. These changes resulted in decreased
platelet aggregation.

　　Adam et al. (1986) and Adam (1987) administered 0, 4, 8,
12, and 16 en% 18:2n-3 with 30 en% from fat to 12 healthy fe-

males for 2 weeks, while another group received 1.7 en% from
EPA. These subjects were receiving 30% of energy as fat at a total
caloric intake of around 2200 kcal. Feeding 18:3n-3 triglycerides
prolonged bleeding time and inhibited platelet aggregation and
prostaglandin synthesis, especially when intake was above 12% of
total energy. A decrease in PGE_2 within 24 hr was observed at a
level of 8 en%. However, feeding 20:5n-3 (EPA) influenced these
parameters by an order of magnitude greater than did 18:3n-3.
The authors conclude that 1.7 en% EPA is sufficient to affect
thrombocyte function in humans. This corresponds to approximately 3 g of EPA per day in normal individuals (around 50 mg/
kg/day). In these diets 18:2n-6 intake was low, at 4 en%. Linolenic acid would have to be ingested at a level at least 5 times as great
as EPA, (i.e., approximately 250 mg/kg body weight/day, to real-
ize comparable trends in the parameters measured. Significantly,
this was at an 18:2 intake level of 4 en%. These data suggest that
dietary linolenic acid has less effect on platelet aggregation than
EPA. However, the data of Renaud (1987) indicate that long-term
ingestion of dietary lipids containing 18:3n-3 acids does affect eicosanoid synthesis, platelet aggregation, and the incidence of thrombosis.

While the metabolic effects of 18:3n-3 may be due mostly to
its elongation products, they can also directly reduce eicosanoid
synthesis by tissues. For example, stimulated mouse macrophages
synthesized 3.0, 2.3, 1.8, 1.6, and 1.5 ng leukotriene B_4 (LTB_4)/
μg cell DNA and 12.7, 13.1, 10.7, 7.5, and 8.7 ng LTC_4/μg DNA,
following ex vivo incubation with 18:2n-6, 18:1n-9, 18:3n-3,
20:5n-3, or 22:6n-3, respectively, indicating effective reduction
of leukotriene synthesis by 18:3n-3. These studies also revealed
the efficacy of DHA in reducing leukotriene synthesis (Lokesh
et al., 1988).

Of the long-chain n-3 PUFAs, EPA appears to be much more
effective than DHA in altering platelet phospholipids, i.e., replacing AA by EPA, suppressing thromboxane, and reducing platelet
aggregability (von Schacky et al., 1985a; Bruckner et al., 1985).
The effects of EPA have been attributed to the synthesis of EPA-
derived eicosanoids, which are less active than those derived from

AA, e.g., TXA_3 vs. TXA_2. However, EPA is a relatively poor substrate for CO, and the principal mechanism by which EPA exerts its antithrombotic activity is by direct competition with AA for cyclooxygenase rather than the formation of PGI_3. Oral ingestion of EPA ethyl ester (3.6 g/day) increased EPA in platelet PL and reduced TXA_2 and platelet aggregability in Japanese subjects (Hirai et al., 1987). Thus, though EPA is a poor substrate for CO in platelets, it competitively inhibits the formation of TXA_2 from AA and reduces aggregability.

Eicosanoids, particularly PGE_2 and LTB_4 are involved in inflammatory reactions (erythema, edema, and hyperalgesia), and LTB_4 also plays an important role in infection and chemotaxis (Gerrard, 1985, Lewis and Flusten, 1984; Bailey, 1986). Thus, agents that inhibit both the CO and lipoxygenase (LO) pathways can have an antiinflammatory effect. EPA is a relatively good substrate for LO, and in monocytes, neutrophils, and macrophages it is efficiently converted by LO to 5-HEPE and LTB_5, which is a much less active chemotactic agent than LTB_4. Thus, EPA, by reducing eicosanoids and LTB_4, offers an approach for modifying inflammatory responses (Lands, 1986; Lee et al., 1985; Goetzl et al., 1986). Terano (1987) reported that supplementation of the normal diet of healthy humans with 3.6 g of EPA day for 4 weeks increased the content of EPA and DPA and decreased the content of AA in PC and PE fractions of neutrophil PL. These changes resulted in a significant reduction in LTB_4 and an increase in LTB_5 upon stimulation of neutrophils. The decreased synthesis of LTB_4 caused by EPA reduces chemotaxis and recruitment of neutrophils and monocytes and suppresses inflammation (Goetzl et al., 1986).

Because fish oils contain significant amounts of DHA, the relative potency of DHA compared to EPA is of interest. In studies with human subjects receiving supplements of 3.6 g/day ethyl esters of EPA or DHA there was no difference in the rate of absorption between DHA and EPA (Hirai et al., 1987). DHA ingestion caused an increase in DHA, and also in EPA content, of plasma phospholipids, whereas AA and docosapentaenoic acid (DPA) showed little change. There was a marked increase in DHA in PC and PE of platelets with little change in AA content. Platelet aggregation induced in vitro by collagen (1 μg/ml) was significantly decreased by DHA ingestion. The EPA was rapidly absorbed and acylated into platelet PC and PE fractions without conversion to DHA. However, significant increases in DPA occurred, indicating that in humans, EPA can readily be elongated to DPA but further desaturation to DHA is apparently limited. In contrast, dietary DHA increased DHA, DPA, and EPA levels in PC and PE fractions of platelets, suggesting retroconversion of DHA. These authors concluded that both EPA and DHA of marine lipids can reduce aggregation of platelets in vitro, though DHA seems to be less potent than EPA (Hirai et al., 1987a,b).

Kobayashi (1987) reporated that a mixture of fish oils containing EPA and DHA decreased platelet aggregation, reduced blood viscosity, and increased red blood cell (RBC) deformability. DHA, from squid oil, was fed at a rate of 3.6 g/day to 12 healthy Japanese subjects and blood was analyzed. Dietary DHA increased EPA from 2 to 3.6% and DHA from 6 to 7.5% of plasma phospholipids after 4 weeks without changing AA levels. While blood viscosity at higher shear rate did not change, RBC deformability increased slightly in these patients (Kobayshi, 1987).

Dietary DHA also affects eicosanoid synthesis in neutrophils. Supplementation of diets with DHA (3.6 g/day) significantly increased human neutrophil DHA and DPA without altering AA. Nevertheless, stimulation of the neutrophils in vitro with ionophore gave significant reductions in LTB_4 formation and an increase in LTB_5 production (Terano, 1987; Hirai et al., 1987a,b). After DHA administration, only LTB_5 production significantly increased. These workers (Terano, 1987; Hirai et al., 1987a,b) concluded that there is limited, if any conversion of EPA to DHA in Japanese subjects, though retroconversion of DHA to EPA may occur. However, this conclusion, based on short-term studies of patients with high endogenous levels of n-3 PUFA, may not be universally valid.

In animal studies, DHA may be selectively incorporated into specific PL in macrophages and specifically reduce LTB_4 synthesis (Lokesh et al., 1988). Overall, the limited data suggest that

EPA and DHA, while having some common general effects, may preferentially affect different AA pools and eicosanoid systems, depending on the tissue or cell type. This possibility requires more study.

INTAKES AND APPROPRIATE DOSAGE OF n-3 PUFA

Eskimos consume approximately 42% calories from fat in a diet of over 3000 kcal. Their diet provides 4.6, 2.6, and 6% EPA, DPA, and DHA, respectively, and about 0.6% 18:3n-3, i.e., a total of 13-14% n-3 PUFA. The diet also contains about 5% 18:2n-6 and 0.4% AA (Dyerberg, 1986). This corresponds to an n-6:n-3 PUFA ratio of 1:3 in the Eskimo diet.

The mean caloric intake in Japan is around 2500 kcals/day, with 500-700 kcal coming from dietary fat, depending on rural or urban lifestyle (Tamura et al., 1986). The average intake of fish is 90 g/day, i.e., corresponding to 1-2 g fat. In fishing villages, seafood intake is around 200 g/day, providing 3-5 g fat and approximately 1 g n-3 PUFA. Because the consumption of visible fats, i.e., vegetable oils, is somewhat limited compared to the U.S. consumption, the n-6:n-3 ratio in the Japanese diet is around 3:1 (Tamura et al., 1986). This is changing, but compares with current values ranging from 15:1 to 50:1 in the United States.

A tentative extrapolation based on the above data might suggest a desirable level of intake of n-3 FA of 3-4 g/day. This is a difficult goal to attain in terms of conventional diet, and significant adjustments might be required in the diet.

SOURCES OF DIETARY n-3 POLYUNSATURATED FATTY ACIDS

Current dietary sources of n-3 PUFA are limited mostly to seafoods, leafy vegetables, marine and some seed oils. Additional potential sources are mentioned below. The most appropriate way to provide n-3 PUFA is as a part of the normal dietary regimen. In this respect, fish and seafoods are the most practical source of n-3 PUFA.

Fish and Seafood Lipids

The world's sustainable yield of fish is around 55 million metric tons per annum, with potentially more from underused species and increasingly from aquaculture (Ackman, 1982; Bimbo, 1987). Of the numerous species available, relatively few species are consumed in the United States, where current consumption at approximately 7 kg per capita per annum is slowly increasing. The major market products are summarized in Table 4. The increased use of underutilized species for engineered fish products (surimi) accounts for some of the expanding consumption (Salvage, 1987).

Fish and seafoods vary immensely in terms of providing n-3 PUFA because of the marked variability in lipid content and fatty acid composition between and within species. The total lipids of fish can range from 1 to 25 g/100 g muscle, but most common species have less than 5% fat (Stansby and Barlow, 1982; Ackman, 1973, 1980, 1982, 1988). The phospholipid, cholesterol, and triglyceride content ranges from 0.4 to 0.7, 0.025 to 0.06, and 1 to 20 g/100 g fish tissue, respectively.

The mean range of fat content in various fish species is summarized in Table 5. Many species commonly consumed, i.e., bass, cod, flounder, haddock, hake, pollock, whiting, skipjack, tuna, scallop, shrimp, clam, trout, and so forth, contain very little fat,

Table 4   Major Seafood Sales in Dollar Value ($ $\times$ 10^6) and Amount (10^6 lb) in United States in 1986

	Dollar value	Amount
Salmon (canned)	245	97
Sardines (canned)	97	35
Tuna (canned)	1425	630
Misc. (canned seafoods)	157	65
Frozen fish (total)	885	283
Fish sticks (breaded)	174	74
Fillets and steaks (breaded)	169	59
Fillets (fresh)	138	45
Frozen crabs	9	1

Table 5   Average Fat Content (mg/100 g Fillet) of Several Common Fish/Seafood

	Percent		Percent		Percent
Low fat		High fat		High fat	
Bass	2.5	Anchovy (pickled)	10	Perch (b,f)	10+
Catfish	3	Albacore tuna	7	Roe	10
Cod	1-2	Bonito tuna	7+	Sablefish	15
Haddock	1	Caviar	15+	Salmon	5-12
Oysters	2	Eel	18	Salmon canned	7-15
Perch yellow	1	Fish cakes (fried)	9	Salmon (Pac.)	9
Pike	1	Flounder, baked	8	Sardines (c) Atl.	24
Pollack	1	Haddock (b, f)	6-8	Shrimp (f)	10
Scallops	0.4	Herring	2	Scallops (f)	8
Shrimp	0.8	Lake trout	8-10	Trout rainbow	6-8
Medium fat		Mackerel	12	Tuna (c, oil)	8-10
Blue fish	5	Menhaden	10	Tuna (c, o, drained)	8-10
Porgy	3	Mullet	7		
Scallops (f)	1-2				
Salmon Pink	4				
Shrimp (4)	1				
Tuna bluefin	4				
Trout	5				

b = baked; f = deep fat fried; c = canned.
Source: Ackman, 1980, 1982.

while salmon, tuna, albacore, bonito, anchovy, herring, mackerel, trout, pilchard, and pompano contain up to 12% fat.

Fish tissue contains approximately 0.5% phospholipids, and the lipids that accumulate beyond this level are mostly triglycerides in most fish species. Fish such as cod, flounder, haddock, and whiting have approximately 1% total triglycerides in their flesh, whereas herring, mackerel, menhaden, and salmon tend to have relatively high levels of triglycerides, depending on the season. The fat in many species of fish exists as a subcutaneous fat layer, though in others the fat is scattered through the muscle. The belly flap and the nape tend to be richer in fat. The dark muscle (lateral line) tends to be richer in lipids and the phospholipid concentration may be 2-3 times that of light muscle (Ackman 1982). Cod and shark accumulate most of their triglycerides in liver rather than in the muscle tissue. Thus, in cod, the oil may account for 80% of the liver mass (which amounts to 10% of the body weight), whereas in herring or salmon, the liver constitutes around 3% of the body weight and contains around 5% fat. Most shellfish have 1-2% fat; crab may have up to 5% and lobster 3.5% fat per edible portion. Triglycerides are the predominant components of fish lipids, though in some species, glyceryl lipids and wax esters may occur (Ackman, 1986). Fatty fish used for edible oil include halibut, mackerel, anchovy, herring, cod, pilchard, capelin, and menhaden, but some of these may also be consumed directly (Stansby and Barlow, 1982; Ackman, 1973, 1980, 1982, 1988).

The triglycerides of fish contain over 50 individual fatty acids, but 8-10 fatty acids usually dominate. The triglycerides contain from 23 to 25% saturated fatty acids and 20 to 35% monenoic fatty acids; the remainder are mostly PUFA. The phospholipids, which amount to approximtely 0.5 g/100 g of wet muscle. ranging from 0.4 to 1.5 for white and dark muscle, respectively, tend to have a higher content of the unsaturated fatty acids which are peculiar to particular species (Table 6). Based on phospholipid content alone, the fatty acid content of fillets is approximately 0.4 g/100 g of muscle. Therefore, assuming that the n-3 PUFAs amount to 30% of these fatty acids, these would provide

Table 6   Relative Amounts (Weight Percent) of n-3 Polyunsaturated Fatty Acids in Triglycerides (TG) and Phospholipids (PL) in Some Fish Species

Fish species	Lipid classes	EPA 20:5	DPA 22:5	DHA 22:6
Cod	TG	17	1.5	26
	PL	15	1.2	32
Sole	TG	10	10	7
	PL	17	9	21
Halibut	TG	13	2.5	37
	PL	8	5	45
Herring	TG	7	t	3
	PL	12	1	32
Salmon Coho	TG	5	4	10
	PL	4	4	10
Dogfish	TG	8	3	21
	PL	5	2	32
Mackerel	TG	8	1.5	13
	PL	10	2.0	36
Shark liver	TG	6	2.0	24
	PL	8	3.0	30
Menhaden	TG	17	2.0	8
	PL	15	3.0	10

EPA = eicosapentaenoic; DPA = docosapentaenoic; DHA = docosahexaenoic acid.
Source: Ackman (1973) and Kinsella et al. (1978).

approximately 90 mg of n-3 PUFA per 100 g (3 oz of fish), a limited source in the contemporary American diet.

In considering fish and seafoods, the wide range and heterogeniety of fatty acids, some of which are unusual, need to be considered. The relatively high amounts of saturated fatty acids (mostly 14:0 and 16:0) in seafoods and fish oil should be recognized (Table 7). In addition, some fish lipids contain high concentrations of monenoic (16:1, 18:1, 20:1, 22:1) fatty acids, e.g., herring vs. pilchard or menhaden lipids. These are unusual components in the U.S. diet. The nutritional implications of these

Table 7   Representative Distribution of Fatty Acids and Cholesterol in Some Common Fatty Fish and Fresh Fish Oils

| | | Fatty acids (Percent) | | | |
Oil	Satd.	Mono-unsatd.	LNA 18:3	EPA 20:5	DHA 22:6	Chol.
Cod liver	18	51	0.7	9.0	9.5	570
Herring	19	60	0.6	7.1	4.3	760
Menhaden	34	32	1.0	12.7	8.0	600
Salmon	24	40	1.0	8.0	11.0	485
Pilchard	25	29	t	17	9.0	—
Mackerel	21	43	t	11	11	—
Anchovy	28	29	t	17	9	—
Sardine	24	34	t	15	10	—

Source: Ackman (1982), Bimbo (1987), Kinsella (1987a).

have been reviewed (Stansby and Barlow, 1982). The n-3 PUFA
components of fish lipids are mostly EPA and DHA with small
amounts of 18:3n-3 (Table 7). Significantly, the sum of these
rarely exceed 20% of the total fatty acids (Ackman, 1982; Hearn
et al., 1987).

The relative concentrations of EPA and DHA differ significantly among species (Table 8), and even within species, marked
variations are noted in concentrations of these fatty acids (Ackman 1982; Kinsella et al., 1978; Hearn et al., 1987). This variability may reflect geographical factors, season of catch, food supply, and so forth, as well as the relative activities of the various
desaturases and elongases in different species of fish.

Because of this variability, specification of a seafood or an
oil according to its source may be inadequate. It is necessary to
provide data on fat content and the EPA and DHA levels. This is
particularly important in clinical trials and/or dietary intervention
regimens. Herring oil is a case in point. It is high in long-chain
fatty acids, but in some samples, these are mostly monoenoic fatty
acids which may account for over 60% of the total fatty acids.
Furthermore, the presence of relatively high concentrations of

Table 8 The Fat and n-3 Polyunsaturated Fatty Acid Content of
Common Fishes and Shellfish (g/100 g Fish)

	Fat	EPA	DHA
Fish			
Blue fish	6.5	0.4	0.8
Capelin	8.2	0.6	0.5
Carp	5.6	0.2	0.1
Catfish	3.7	0.2	0.2
Cod (Atlantic)	1.0	0.1	0.2
Dogfish	10.0	0.7	1.2
Flounder	1.0	0.1	0.1
Grouper	0.8	t	0.2
Haddock	0.7	0.1	0.1
Hake	0.6	t	t
Halibut	13.8	0.5	0.4
Herring	10.0	1.0	0.9
Mackerel	13.0	1.0	1.6
Perch (ocean)	1.5	0.1	0.1
Plaice	1.5	0.1	0.1
Pollock	1.0	0.1	0.4
Pompano	9.5	0.2	0.4
Salmon (Atl)	5.4	0.3	0.9
Salmon (Chinook)	10.5	0.8	0.7
Salmon (Coho)	6.0	0.3	0.5
Salmon (sockeye)	8.6	0.5	0.7
Sheepshead	2.4	0.1	0.1
Smelt (rainbow)	2.6	0.3	0.4
Snapper (red)	1.2	t	0.2
Sole	1.2	t	0.1
Swordfish	2.1	0.1	0.1
Trout (char)	7.7	0.1	0.5
Trout (lake)	9.7	0.5	1.1
Trout (rainbow)	3.4	0.1	0.4
Tuna (albacore)	5.0	0.3	1.0
Tuna (bluefish)	6.6	0.4	1.2
Tuna (skipjack)	1.9	0.1	0.3
Whiting	0.5	t	0.1

Table 8 (continued)

	Fat	EPA	DHA
Crustaceans			
Crab (Alaska)	0.8	0.2	0.1
Crab (Blue)	1.3	0.2	0.2
Crayfish	1.4	0.1	t
Lobster	1.0	0.1	0.1
Shrimp	1.5	0.2	0.2
Spiny lobster	1.4	0.2	0.1
Mollusks			
Clam	0.7	0.1	0.1
Mussel	2.2	0.2	0.3
Octopus	1.0	0.1	0.1
Oyster	2.3	0.3	0.2
Scallop	0.8	0.1	0.1
Squid	1.5	0.1	0.2

$C14:0$ in menhaden oil should be recognized. Data concerning the fatty acid composition of seafood lipids and factors affecting it have been extensively reviewed and compiled by Ackman (1982) and Barlow and Stansby (1982).

Sinclair et al. (1986) reported on the widely differing fatty acid composition of fish caught around Australia. Generally, fish caught in warm water around latitudes 10-12° south contained low levels of lipids (1-2%) but significant amounts of arachidonic acid, i.e., 10-16% with a total n-6 PUFA level of 19-26%, while EPA ranged from 2 to 5% and DHA from 26 to 30% depending on the species. This was in contrast to Antarctic fish, which contained varying amounts of fat (1-2%), limited AA (1-2%) (though some had up to 25%), up to 30% EPA, and up to 52% DHA. Generally, Antarctic fish are much richer in DHA than in EPA. These data indicated that the fish caught closer to the equator have higher levels of AA. Based on these data, one cannot make a universal statement that fish consumption ensures a supply of n-3 PUFA. In studies with five healthy males consumption of 500 g of samples of these fish per day for 2 weeks (32 en% from fat) caused significant changes in plasma acids within 7 days (Sinclair et al., 1986). Tropical fish rich in AA and DHA increased the 18:2n-6 levels in plasma phospholipids with modest increases in AA and DHA levels in these lipids. The rise in plasma AA in subjects on a tropical fish was consistently associated with an increased platelet thromboxane production in vitro. These studies underline the need to determine carefully fatty acid composition of fish used in the diet. Kinsella et al. (1978) and Hearn et al. (1987) showed that certain freshwater species, e.g., pike contain significant amounts of n-6 PUFA such as 20:4n-6.

In the context of n-3 consumption the summary data (Table 8) are of practical value for estimating the amount of EPA and DHA available from some common fish and shellfish.

Much of the available data are based on analyses of raw fish, and while some cooking methods cause negligible changes (especially for low-fat fish) (Table 9), the method of preparation, medium, and method of cooking can result in significant changes (Mai et al., 1978; Kinsella 1987b). Thus, when discussing fish as a component of the diet, particularly as a source of n-3 PUFA, it should be remembered that a large proportion of the fish consumed in the United States consists of breaded portions, much of which is deep-fat fried. The fat content of breaded fish fillets, fish sticks,

Table 9   Changes in Fatty Acids of Trout Fillets (7% Fat) Following Cooking by Different Methods (mg/100 g Fillet)

Fatty acids	Raw	Baked	Raw	Pan-fried	Raw	Deep fried
Satd. FA	1233	1012	1424	1535	1237	1283
Monoenes	2506	1991	3203	3507	1844	2796
18:2 n6	244	192	528	354	505	277
20:4 n6	232	195	285	327	198	253
20:5 n3	330	282	404	468	327	371
22: n6	800	760	980	1001	920	1024
Total FA	6229	5110	7843	8391	6710	6805

Source: Mai et al. (1978).

and so on, may range from 3 to 20% fat, which is composed mostly of the cooking oil (Nettleton, 1985; Ackman, 1982). Ironically, many of the fish sticks are made from cod, which normally contains around 1% lipid material.

The physiological effects of n-3 PUFA depend on the relative concentration of fat in the diet, particularly of n-6 polyunsaturated fatty acids. The fat content and composition of many seafood items are determined by the cooking oil. Thus, whereas steamed cod may contain around 1% lipids, this increases to 5% following frying; flounder steamed and fried has around 2 and 12% fat, respectively; haddock steamed and fried contains 1 and 8% fat; herring raw and fried about 18% and 15% fat; i.e., in high-fat species, cooking may cause a reduction in fat content; lemon sole steamed and fried has 1 and 13%, respectively; plaice steamed and fried has 2 and 14% fat (Ackman, 1973). Smoking of fish results in a relative increase in fat, which reflects the concomitant dehydration. Thus, halibut, with 4.5% fat in the fresh state, contains about 15% fat following smoking; herring increases from 10 to 14% (Ackman, 1973). Canned fish, e.g., tuna and salmon, may have a very variable fat content depending on whether it is canned in vegetable oil or water.

Freshwater fish contain significant amounts of n-3 PUFA; e.g., lake trout, rainbow trout, and pike contain, respectively, 40, 27, and 30% EPA plus DHA and thus could be good sources of these fatty acids. Incidentally, these fish also contain considerable amounts of n-6 PUFA (Kinsella et al., 1978). Fish raised by aquacultural methods contain n-3 PUFA (Table 10), but generally in a lower quantity than in the corresponding free-living species because the concentrations of n-3 and n-6 PUFA tend to reflect the lipids in the diet (Suzuki et al., 1986; Chanmugam et al., 1986). Cultured eel contains significant amounts of n-3 PUFA, i.e., 35% and 10% in PL and triglycerides, respectively (Otwell and Richards, 1982).

In considering fish as a source of n-3 PUFA, excess intake of cholesterol does not appear to be a significant problem. Fish fillets contain 30-60 mg cholesterol per 100 g. Thus, 100 g tuna, which provides approximately 0.5 g n-3 PUFA, delivers around 35

Table 10 Fatty Acid Composition of Lipids of Cultured and "Wild" Fish

	Carp		Trout		Catfish	
Fatty acids	Cultured	Wild	Cultured	Wild	Cultured	Wild
Saturated	19.0	29.0	32.1	30.9	26.6	28.0
16:1 n7	7.4	8.1	3.7	9.5	4.1	7.0
18:2 n6	15.2	6.0	16.6	21.6	12.5	3.0
18:3 n3	1.1	1.8	1.0	7.0	1.7	2.7
20:4 n6	1.0	7.5	1.5	1.7	1.8	6.8
20:5 n3	2.5	7.0	5.2	5.3	1.5	7.0
22:6 n3	6.0	7.0	26.0	11.7	5.0	13.5

Source: Suzuki et al. (1986), Chanmugam et al. (1986).

mg cholesterol, while 100 g salmon provides 1.5 g n-3 PUFA and approximately 60 mg cholesterol. Shellfish, which are low in fat and n-3 PUFA, may contain higher levels of cholesterol (Nettleton, 1985).

A diet consistently containing certain species of fatty fish, e.g., salmon, tuna, and trout, with limited amounts of visible fats should provide adequate quantities of n-3 PUFA.

EDIBLE OILS CONTAINING n-3 PUFA

While this chapter is concerned with marine sources of fatty acids, it should be noted that some vegetable oils, e.g., linseed, rapeseed (canola), and soybean oils, containing 55, 10, and 7% alpha linolenic acid (18:3n-3), respectively, are produced in large volumes worldwide (Table 11).

World production of fish oils is approximately 1.5×10^6 metric tons, of which 0.14×10^6 metric tons is produced in the United States (Bimbo, 1987). The preponderance of commercial fish oil is extracted from fatty fish [e.g., menhaden (United States), anchovy (Peru), sardine (Japan), capelin, herring, mackerel, sand eel, pilchard]; some from fish liver, especially cod and

Table 11   World Production[a] of Oils Containing n-3 Polyunsaturated Fatty Acids (Metric Ton 10^3)

	Total oil	Estimated n-3 PUFA
Soybean	14,000	640
Rapeseed	6,250	600
Linseed	600	380
Butterfat	5,400	54
Marine oil[b]	1,500	300

[a]USDA Oilseeds and Products Reports, 1986.
[b]FAO Yearbook Fishery Statistics, 1984.

some shark; and small quantities from fish scraps and by-products
(Bimbo, 1987). The major fish oil-producing nations are Norway,
Japan, Peru, and the United States. Most fish oil is used in Britain,
Norway, Peru, Germany, and the Netherlands as shortening and
margarine. The consumption in the United States is negligible
(Young, 1982; Bimbo, 1987).

The fatty acid (FA) composition of fish oils (Tables 12 and
13) varies with the species from which they are derived. Generally, menhaden and pilchard oils contain relatively high levels of
EPA, and this, together with DHA (which is the major n-3 PUFA
in many fish) rarely exceeds 25% of the total FA. Thus, in selecting a fish oil the other fatty acid components, i.e., the amounts of
saturated fatty acids (palmitic and myristic acid), and the quantities of long-chain monoenoic acids are of concern. In addition,
the concentrations of cholesterol, vitamins A and D, pesticides,
and tocopherol in various oils are of practical and safety interest
(Kinsella, 1987a).

Currently, several fish oils are available in bulk or in encapsulated refined form. These are derived mostly from menhaden,
sardine, or cod liver oils, though mackerel, herring, anchovy, pilchard, tuna, and salmon oils may be used if available.

Care must be exercised in selecting capsules to ensure the appropriate n-3 PUFA and tocopherol contents, low levels of choles-

Table 12 Fatty Acid Composition of Some Fish Oils

Fatty acids	Menhaden	Cod liver	Shark liver	Rainbow trout liver
14:0	8.0	1.1	0.9	8.7
16:0	24.2	18.5	15.9	18.2
16:1	10.5	3.7	2.3	13.8
18:0	3.0	5.3	9.4	5.5
18:1	23.4	14.7	18.9	13.9
18:2 (LA)	2.1	1.7	4.1	3.4
20:1	1.8	9.8	4.1	1.8
22:0	2.0	4.2	2.3	1.6
22:1	1.6	2.3	1.6	3.4
20:4 n6 (AA)	2.1	0.4	4.1	1.2
20:5 n3 (EPA)	14.0	6.4	4.3	15.5
22:6 n3 (DHA)	11.6	27.4	30.0	7.0

Table 13 Range in Fatty Acid Composition of Herring and Menhaden Oils

Fatty acid	Herring		Menhaden	
	Maximum	Minimum	Maximum	Minimum
14:0	8	5	16	7
16:0	15	10	24	19
16:1	12	6	18	11
18:1	21	9	23	10
20:1	20	11	2	t
22:1	31	15	t	t
20:5	9	4	18	10
22:6	6	2	12	4

Source: Data from Stansby and Barlow (1982); Kinsella (1987a).

terol, and the absence of pesticide residues. In some preparations, the amounts of n-3 PUFA may be overestimated; e.g., a recent sampling of commercial encapsulated fish oils revealed from 18 to 35% EPA and 11 to 19% DHA (Anon., 1987). Cholesterol may range from 10 to 500 mg/100 g, and in the case of liver oils, the levels of vitamin A and D can be very high (Kinsella, 1987a). Most commercial products from reputable manufacturers have been refined and distilled to remove the undesirable components and reliably meet label claims.

Digestion

Dietary polyunsaturated fats are readily digested, absorbed, and incorporated in lipoproteins (Herold and Kinsella, 1986; Nelson and Ackman, 1988; Chen et al., 1985). Dietary n-3 PUFAs are interconverted at relatively slow rates in humans. There is some evidence that dietary DHA may be retroconverted to EPA in humans (Hirai et al., 1987) though the extent and significance of this are unknown. The n-3 PUFAs of dietary fish oils are readily incorporated into membranes, though the relative rates and extent of uptake of EPA and DHA vary with tissue (Swanson et al., 1987, 1988). Thus platelets show a preference for EPA (Bruckner et al., 1985), whereas cardiac and other tissues selectively incorporate DNA DNA (Salem, 1986; Swanson et al., 1987).

The dosage of fish oils required to cause hypolipidemic effects varies with n-3 PUFA content and n-6 content of the diet. However, salmon oil at 30 ml/day (approximately 5 g n-3 PUFA per day) is effective (Connor, 1986), and menhaden oil is reported to be effective at intakes ranging from 10 to 20 g/day, i.e., 2-4 g n-3 PUFA (Saynor et al., 1986). Other oils (cod liver, sardine, squid) are also effective at relatively high dosages, e.g., 30-40 ml/day (von Schacky et al., 1986; Knapp et al., 1986). Continual ingestion is required for sustained effects (Saynor et al., 1986).

PROCESSING AND FRACTIONATION OF FISH OILS

Hydrogenation

Most of the marine oils produced worldwide are hydrogenated for use in margarines, shortenings, and frying oils, in Europe. Hydrogenation improves the physical properties and plastic/melting range of the oils, and by elimination of the double bonds, it improves stability (Ackman 1982; Bimbo, 1987). Lightly hydrogenated marine oils with iodine values around 120 are liquid and are useful in salad oils or for use in shallow frying. These contain about 4 and 3% EPA and DHA, respectively (Sebedio and Ackman, 1986). For most margarine and shortening uses, marine oils are hydrogenated to iodine values below 90, where they are mostly plastic and used for shortening applications. These have negligible quantities of n-3 PUFA (Stansby, 1976).

Fractionation of Fish Oils

To minimize overall fat intake and to obviate some problems in terms of flavor, smell, eructative unpleasantness, and so on, it may be desirable to fractionate fish oils to produce edible oils or capsules containing mostly concentrated n-3 PUFA. This would effectively reduce the amount of oil required (three to fourfold) and greatly facilitate compliance with intervention and supplementation regimens.

The fractionation of fish oils is difficult because of the marked heterogeneity in fatty acid composition, particularly in the range of unsaturated fatty acid components of fish oils. Generally, the content of n3 PUFA amounts to 15-30% of total fatty acids. Second, many of the fatty acids have 20 carbon chains, which makes it difficult to separate monoenoic from polyeonic fatty acids with a reasonable degree of purification. Many efforts have been made to produce EPA-enriched oils with low levels of DPA and DHA. For a putative antithrombotic effect, it may be desirable to provide oils that have high EPA concentrations because platelets apparently preferentially absorb EPA at the expense of arachidonic acid. DHA appears to be as effective as EPA in suppressing leukotriene synthesis by macrophages (Lokesh et al., 1988). These two observations underscore the need to define the function of different n-3 PUFAs because conceivably, depending on the desired effect, different preparations may be desirable for different applications. Further research should elucidate this question.

Several methods have been explored for fractionating fish oils to obtain n-3 PUFA-rich fractions (Ackman, 1986). Since most of these methods are based on physical properties such as molecular size, vapor pressure, and so on, it is difficult to separate EPA, DPA, and DHA. Many of the methods used for fractionation of fish oils require large volumes of solvents, and generally yields are quite low. A number of methods exploiting solvent partitioning have been used; these have been briefly discussed by Ackman (1986).

Molecular Distillation

Molecular distillation can be effective for the preparation of omega-3 PUFA from fish oils, particularly as their ethyl or methyl esters.

Fractional Crystallization

Certain fish oils tend to be high in saturated and monoenoic fatty acids. These include herring, capelin, cod liver, anchovy, pilchard, menhaden, and whale oil (Ackman, 1986). These oils also tend to be higher in polyunsaturated fatty acids. Therefore, simple fractional crystallization (winterization), directly or from solvents, can provide a modest increase in the n-3 PUFA glycerides. Thus, Ackman (1986) reported an increase from 18 to 25% in n-3 PUFA following winterization of menhaden oil at 8°C. Winterization at −18°C and −35°C from acetone increased the n-3 PUFA to 26 and 30%, respectively, with yields of 87 and 70%. The use of esters of fatty acids, which accentuate differences in physical properties, improves the yields from fractional crystallization and countercurrent solvent/solvent partitioning. Countercurrent fractionation coupled with crystallization of free acids or esters can increase n-3 PUFA concentrations by up to 50% (Ackman, 1986).

Vacuum Distillation

Vacuum distillation can be effectively used to remove saturated fatty acids and some monoenoic fatty acids from fish oil fatty acid mixes.

Urea Fractionation

Urea complex formation of fatty acids has been extensively used for enriching fish oils in n-3 PUFA (Stout, 1963). Urea fractionation of the fatty acids from ethanol or methanol can give fractions containing 50-60% n-3 PUFA and up to 30% EPA from menhaden oil fatty acids in yields averaging 30% (Ackman, 1986). Recrystallization from urea three times provided the most effective enrichment of 60%. When urea crystallization was used after countercurrent fractionation, an enrichment up to 56% n-3 PUFA at a yield of 66% was obtained. Repetition of this sequence further improved the enrichment in n-3 PUFA (Olsson, 1984). Thus, it appears that urea crystallization is a practical method amenable to scale and yielding up reasonable quantities of n-3 PUFA. Prior saponification facilitates the removal of sterols, vitamins A and D, xenobiotics (PCB), and other undesirable components from the oil. Urea fractionation of lithium soaps is effective in concentrating DHA from fish oils (Bruckner et al., 1985). Haagsma et al. (1982) described a urea fractionation method for enriching the EPA and DHA levels of cod liver oil from 12 to 28 and 11 to 45%, respectively.

Supercritical Fractionation

Supercritical fractionation of fish oils using supercritical CO_2 (SCO_2) can be effective in preparing enriched fractions of n-3 PUFA. This method is mild and, because it uses CO_2, minimizes autooxidation. It separates most effectively on the basis of chain length; hence the method works best for oils with a low level of 20-carbon monoenoic fatty acids. Esters of fatty acids are more effectively fractionated by SCO_2 than triglycerides. This method has been effectively used to refine fish oils and remove cholesterol, PCBs, vitamin E, and other components (Daniels et al., 1988).

A number of oils enriched in n-3 PUFAs are currently available with 30, 50, and up to 90% EPA. These are generally prepared by fractional crystallization, urea adduct separation, or distillation. A large number (15-20) of pharmaceutical companies are now marketing encapsulated refined and enriched fish oils with added tocopherol, for stability. These are widely available in health food stores though they have not been approved by the Food and Drug Administration. The British preparation maxEPA was recently approved for clinical applications in the United Kingdom.

OTHER SOURCES OF n-3 PUFA

Ultimately, n-3 PUFAs are derived from photosynthetic autotrophs, i.e., algae and plants. Photosynthetic tissue, i.e., chloroplasts in higher plants, contain high levels of linolenic acid 18:3n-3 (45-70%) mostly in the galactosylglycerolipids. The leaves of higher plants contain 5-8% total lipids, mostly polar lipids galactosyl- and phosphoglycerides (Hitchcock and Nichols, 1971). The 18:2n-6:18:3n-3 ratio in plant leaves ranges from 0.25 to 0.3. Hence leafy vegetables, lettuce, cabbage, turnip greens, spinach, and other vegetables are good sources of 18:3n-3 which may be effective in low-fat diets.

In contrast to photosynthetic tissue, the storage organs (fruits, seeds, nuts) of plants tend to accumulate other fatty acids, mostly 18:3n-6 in the case of oilseeds (Table 14). The exception is linseed (flaxseed) with 56-60% 18:3n-3, some rapeseed cultivars (canola) with 10-14%, and soybean with 6-8% 18:3n-3. Certain nuts and seeds contain high amounts of 18:3n-3 (Table 14). However, most seeds and nuts, with the exception of linseed oil, represent marginal sources of n-3 PUFA and as part of an overall diet are not direct sources of concentrated 18:3n-3. Flaxseed represents a copious source of 18:3n-3 that is used mostly as a base for paints/varnishes. Small amounts of flaxseed are used as a food ingredient in breads. With improved processing and refining, coupled with effective antioxidant use, that linseed oil could become a practical source of dietary n-3 PUFA.

Table 14   The Major Unsaturated Fatty Acids in Vegetable Oils,
Nuts, and Seeds

Oil	Fatty acids (%)		
	18:1n9	18:2n6	18:3n3
Soybean	38	50-60	7.0
Canola	55	24	11.0
Corn	25	60	0.5
Sunflower	20	70	0.5
Safflower	—	70	t
Linseed	20	12	53.0
Walnut	23	50	10.0
Wheatgerm	15	55	7.0
Rice bran	40	35	1.6
Beechnut	23	20	1.8
Butternut	10	32	8.7
Hickory	32	20	1.0
Walnut (black)	13	36	4.0
Currant seed	—	5	3.0

While there appears to be an adequate supply of n-3 PUFA
from fish oil, there is growing interest in nonfish sources, especially algae, which can be grown universally and are amenable to
genetic manipulation (Richmond, 1986). Many algae accumulate
high levels of n-3 PUFA, i.e., EPA or DHA, during growth (Table
15), and because these may contain up to 10% of their biomass as
lipid, they have the potential to become a significant source of
n-3 PUFA. Some species, e.g., *Phacodactyllium* and *Chlorella*,
contain mostly EPA (approximately 30%), while *Gonyaulax* has
mostly DHA (34%) (Sargent, 1976; Seito et al., 1984). The content of these fatty acids may be altered by culture conditions
(Seito et al., 1984). These lipids may be extracted and refined
with supercritical carbon dioxide. Alternatively, dried algae may
be used as a food ingredient. Finally, krill, with 17% lipids in the
dry weight and 15% n-3 PUFA, may be a potential source of n-3
PUFA (Yamaguchi et al., 1986).

Table 15   The n-3 Polyunsaturated Fatty Acid Content of Some Algae

Species	Fatty acid (wt %)		
	LNA 18:3	EPA 20:5	DHA 22:6
Chlorella officinale	2.5	32.0	t
Chlorella minutissima	t	44.0	t
Phaeodactylum tricornutum	t	26.0	11.0
Gonyaulox caterella	1.3	11.2	34.0

Within the immediate future marine oils represent the most practical source of n-3 PUFA. Based on the worldwide production of around 1.5×10^6 metric tons of fish oil, approximately 3×10^5 metric tons of n-3 PUFA are available as components of marine oils. Hence, if fish oil becomes a universal dietary component or even if supplementation becomes more popular, the market will exceed current supply and additional marine, algal, and plant sources of n-3 PUFA will need to be developed.

CONCLUSIONS

The available data suggest that n-3 PUFA may have positive effects on the course of several chronic human diseases (Lands, 1986; Kinsella, 1987a; Leaf and Weber, 1988). Dietary intervention using fish or fish oils as food components, cooking oils, or supplements could be a very attractive prophylactic approach to these diseases. The idea that enriched fish oil preparations may have therapeutic value has excited great interest, as evidenced by commercial developments and promotion. However, accompanying the general optimism some caution is advisable, since eicosanoids, which are derived from PUFA, perform very different, but important functions in many tissues (Gerrard, 1985). The susceptibility of n-3 PUFA to peroxidation and polymerization should be of concern and underscore the need for caution in their use and the potential need for the addition of antioxidants to the diet.

Furthermore, in discussing the effects of n-3 PUFA on eicosanoid production by tissues, the effects observed using in vitro or ex vivo tests or observations from animal studies may not necessarily reflect the in vivo situation in humans where numerous physiological and metabolic control factors are operational. Therefore, in making extrapolations from data derived from in vitro or animal experiments, extreme care mut be exercised, particularly when considering dietary intervention.

The consumption of high levels of n-3 PUFA may prolong bleeding time and cause epitaxis, spontaneous bruising of tissues, and reduction of blood platelet and perhaps erythrocyte counts. The ominous suggestion of Gudbjarnsson et al. (1978) that the accumulation of DHA may sensitize heart muscle to catecholamines and result in sudden death needs to be studied further.

The apparent desirability of maintaining an adequate dietary supply of n-3 PUFA offers an opportunity and a challenge to the food industry. Progress toward this goal could be achieved most simply by increasing fish and seafood consumption and green vegetables. However, considerable improvement in the quality (odor, flavor, taste) of seafoods is still needed to make this approach more attractive. In addition, the food industry may want to explore novel methods for including fish oils and n-3 PUFA rich oilseeds in formulated foods. Success in this area depends on innovative methods for controlling oxidation of the n-3 PUFA. This is the major problem limiting the use of fish oils and warrants more dedicated research.

ACKNOWLEDGEMENT

This work was supported in part by New York Sea Grant Program.

REFERENCES

Ackman RG. Marine lipids and fatty acids in human nutrition. Proc. FAO Tech Conference FAO, Rome, 1973.

Ackman RG, Connel J, ed. Advances in fish science and technology. England: Fishing News Books, 1980:86.

Ackman RG. In: Barlow S, Stansby ME, eds. Nutritional evaluation of fatty acids in fish oil. New York: Academic Press, 1982:25.

Ackman R. Scandanavian lipid-forum for lipid research and technology Report #33, 1986.

Ackman R. Food Technol 42:151, 1988.

Ackman RG, Lamothe M, Hulan H, Proudfoot FG. n-3 News 1988;3(1):1.

Ackman RG, Tarnayake W, Olsson B. J Am Oil Chem Soc 1988; 65(1):37.

Adam O, Wolfram G, Zollner N. Ann Nutr Metab 1986;30:274.

Adam O. In: Lands WE, ed. Polyunsaturated fatty acids and eicosanoids. Champaign, IL: Am Oil Chem Soc, 1987:215.

Ahrens EH, Insull W, Hirsch J, Stoffel W, Peterson M, Miller T, Thompson M. Lancet 1959;1:115.

Anon. J Am Oil Chem Soc 1987;64.

Avery-Nelson M. Geriatrics 1972;27:103.

Bailey M. Prostglandins, leukotrienes and lipoxins. New York: Plenum Press, 1986.

Barlow SM, Stansby ME. Nutritional evaluation of long-chain fatty acids in fish oil. New York: Academic Press, 1982.

Bimbo AP. J Am Oil Chem Soc. 1987;64:206.

Bjerve KS, Thoresen L, Levold-Mostad L, Alme K, Advances PG. Thromboxane Leukotriene 1987a;17:862.

Bjerve K, Levold-Mostad L, Thoresen L. Am J Clin Nutr 1987b; 45:66.

Bronte-Stewart B, Antonis A, Eales L, Brock J. Lancet 1956;1: 521.

Bruckner G, German B, Lokesh B, Kinsella JE. Thrombosis Res 1985;34:479.

Budowski P, Crawford M. Proc Nutr Soc 1985;44:221.

Chanmugam P, Boundreau M, Hwang DH. J Food Sci 1986;51: 1556.

Chen IS, Subramanian S, Cassidy MM, Sheppard AJ, Vanouny JG. J Nutr 1985;115:219.

Connor WE. In: Simopoulos A et al., eds. Health effects of polyunsaturated fatty acids in seafoods. New York: Academic Press 1986.

Connor WE, Witcak DT, STone B, Armstrong MJ. Clin Invest 1969;48:1363.

Daggy B. Arost C, Bensadoun A. Biochim Biophys Acta 1987; 920:293.

Daniels J, Rizvi S, Black J, German B. J Food Sci 1987.

Dyerberg J. Nutr Rev 1986;44;125.

Dyerberg J, Bang H, Hjorne N. Am J Clin Nutr 1975;28:958.

Eaton SB, Konner M. N Engl J Med 1985;312:283.

Flier J, Lokesh B, Kinsella JK. Nutr Res 1985;5:277.

German B, Lokesh B, Kinsella JE. Prost Leukotr Med 1988;34,37.

Gerrard JM. Prostaglandins and leukotrienes. New York: Marcel Dekker, 1985.

Goetzl EJ, Wong M, Paran P, Rogan T. Pickett W, Blake V. In: Simopoulos A, Kifer R, Martin R, eds. Health effects of polyunsaturated fatty acids in seafoods. New York: Academic Press, 1986;239.

Gudbjarnsson S, Oscarsdottier G, Doell B, Halligrimsson. Adv Cardiol 1978;25:130.

Haagsma N, Gent CM, Luten JB, DeJong R, Van Doorn E. J Am Chem Soc 1982;59:117.

Harris WS. J Lipid Res 1989;30:785.

Harris WS, Connor W, McMurrary M. Metabolism 1983;32:179.

Hearn TL, Sgoutos S, Hearn J, Sgoutas D. J Food Sci 1987;52: 1209.

Herold P, Kinsella JE. Am J Clin Nutr 1986;43:560.

Hirai A, Terano T, Takenaga M. Adv Prostgl Thromb Leukotr Res 1987a;17:838.

Hirai A, Terano T, Saito H, Tamura Y, Yoshida S. In: Lands WE, ed. Polyunsaturated fatty acids and eicosanoids. Champaign, IL: Am Oil Chem Soc Press, 1987b; 9.

Hitchcock C, Nichols BW. Plant lipid biochemistry. New York: Academic Press, 1971.

Holman RT. Prog Lipid Res 1986;25:29.

Holman RT, Johnson SB. Nutr Rev 1982;40:144.

Holman RT, Johnson S, Hatch TF. Am J Clin Nutr 1982;35:617.

Hwang DH, Boudreau M, Chanmugam P. J Nutr 1988;118:427.

Iritani N, Inoguchi K, Fukudu E, Moreta M. Biochim Biophys Acta 1980;618:378.

Jacotot B, Lasser M, Mendy F. Prog Lipid Res 1986;25:185.

Kagawa Y, Nishizawa M, Suzuki M, Miyatake T, Hamamoto T, Goto K, Izumikawa H, Hirata H, Ebihara HJ. Nutr Sci Vitaminol 1982;28:441.

Kinsell LW, Michaels G, Walker G, Visintine RE. Diabetes 1961; 10:316.

Kinsella JE. Seafoods and fish oils in human health and disease. New York: Marcel Dekker, 1987a.

Kinsella JE. Am J Cardiol 1987b;60:23G.

Kinsella JE. Food Technol 1988;42:124.

Kinsella JE, Shimp J, Mai J, Weihrauch J. J Am Oil Chem Soc 1977;54:429.

Kinsella JE, Posati L, Weihrauch J. Crit Rev Food Sci Nutr 1975; 5:299.

Kinsella JE, Shimp J, Mai J. NY Food Life Sci Bull. Cornell University #69, 1978.

Kinsella JE, German B, Swanson J, Lokesh B. In: Lands WE, ed.

Polyunsaturated fats and eicosanoids. Champaign, IL:
Amer Oil Chem. Soc., 1987; 416.

Knapp H, Reilly I, FitzGerald G. N Engl J Med 1986;314:937.

Kobayashi Y. Adv Prost Thromb Leukotr Res 1987;17(6):40.

Lands WEM. Polyunsaturated fats and eicosanoids. Champaign,
IL: Am. Oil Chem. Soc., 1987.

Lands WE, Kulmacz RJ. Prog Lipid Res 1986;25:105.

Lands WEM, Letellier P, Rome LH, Vanderhoek J. Adv Biosci
1973;9:15.

Lands WEM. Fish and human health. New York: Academic
Press, 1986.

Leaf A, Weber P. N Engl J Med 1988;73:889..

Lee T, Hover R, Williams J, Sperling R, Robinson D. N Engl J
Med 1985;312:1217.

Lokesh B, German B, and Kinsella JE. Lipids 1988;23:968.

Lokesh B, German B, Kinsella JE. Biochim Biophys Acta 1988;
99:958.

Mai J, Weihrauch J, Kinsella JE. J Food Sci 1978;43:1669.

Naughton J, O'Dea K, Sinclair HA. Lipids 1986;21:11.

Nelson GJ, Ackman RG. Lipids 1988;23:1005.

Nestel PJ. Am J Clin Nutr 1986;43:752.

Nestel P, Wont S, Topping D. In: Kifer R, Martin R, eds. Health
effects of polyunsaturated fatty acids in seafoods. New
York: Academic Press, 1986; 211.

Nettleton J. Seafood nutrition. Huntington, New York: Osprey
Books, 1985.

Neuringer M, Connor WE. Nutr Rev 1986;44:28.

Nikkari T. Prog Lipid Res 1986;25:437.

Nilsson WB, Gauglitz E, Hudson J, Stout VF, Spinelli J. J Am
Oil Chem Soc 1988;65:109.

Olsson B. M.S. thesis. Technical Unit., Nova Scotia, 1984.

Otwell WS, Rickards WL. Aquaculture 1982;26:67.

Phillipson B, Rothrock DW, Connor WE, Harris W, Ellingworth R. N Engl J Med 1985;312:1210.

Quadt J, TenHoor F. Prog Lipid Res 1982;30:581.

Renaud S. In: Lands W, ed. Polyunsaturated fatty acids and eicosanoids. Champaign, IL: Am Oil Chem Soc., 1987; 56.

Richmond AF. CRC Crit Rev Biotech 1986;4:369.

Robertson T, Kato H, Rhoads B. Am J CArdiol 1977;39:239.

Salem N. In: Simopoulos A, ed. Health effects of dietary poly-unsaturated fatty acids in seafoods. New York: Academic Press, 1986.

Salo MK. Prog Lipid Res 1986;25:471.

Salvage V. Prepared Foods, April 1987; 156.

Sanders T, Sullivan D, Reeve J, Sampson J. Atherosclerosis 1985; 5:459.

Sargent JR. Biochem Biophys Perspect Marine Biol 1976;3:100.

Saynor R, Gilott T, Doyle T, Allen D, Field P, Scott M. Prog Lipid Res 1986;25:211.

Sebedio JL, Ackman RG. J Am Oil Chem Soc 1986;60.

Seito A, Want HL, Hesseltin C. J Am Oil Chem Soc 1984;6(1): 892.

Simopoulos A, Kifer P, Martin R. Health effects of dietary poly-unsaturated fatty acids in seafoods. New York: Academic Press, 1986.

Sinclair AJ, O'Dea J, Smith I, Parkin D. Prog Lipid Res 1986; 25:83.

Sprecher H. Prog Lipid Res 1986;25:19.

Stansby M, Barlow ME. Nutritional evaluation of long chain fatty acids in fish oils. New York: Academic Press, 1982.

Stansby ME. Industrial fishery technology. Huntington, New York: Kreiger Publ. Co., 1976.

Stout V. J Am Oil Chem Soc 1963;40:40.

Suzuki H, Okazaki K, Hayakawa S, Wadi S, Tamura S. J Agr Food Chem 1986;34:58.

Swanson J, Black M, Kinsella JE. J Nutr 1987;117:824.

Swanson J, Lokesh B, Kinsella JE. Br J Nutr 1988;59:535.

Tamura Y, Hirai A, Terano T, Saitohn O, Tahara K, Yoshida S. Prog Lipid Res 1986;25:461.

Terano T. Adv PG Thromb Leukotr Res 1987;17:880.

Terano T. Seya A, Saito H, Tamura Y, Yoshida S. In: Lands WE, ed. Polyunsaturated fatty acids and eicosanoids. Champaign, IL: Am. Oil Chem. Soc. Press, 1987; 133.

Tinoco M. Prog Lipid Res 1982;21:1.

von Schacky P, Weber P. J Clin Invest 1985a;76:2446.

von Schacky C, Fischer S, Weber P. J Clin Invest 1985b;76:1626.

Wertz PW. Prog Lipid Res 1986;25:383.

Wong S, Nestel PJ. Atherosclerosis 1987;64:139.

Yamagucchi K, Murakami M, Nakano H, Konosu S, Kokura T, Yamoto H, Kosaka M, Hata K. J Agric Food Chem 1986; 34:904.

Yamori Y, Nara Y, Itiani N, Irigami T. J Nutr Sci Vitamin 1985; 321:417.

Young FVK. In: Barlow SM, Stansby ME, eds. Nutritional evaluation of long-chain fatty acidsin fish oils. New York: Academic Press, 1982; 1.

Zollner N. Prog Lipid Res 1986;25:177.

8
Supercritical Fluid Fractionation of Fish Oils

Val Krukonis
Phasex Corporation
Lawrence, Massachusetts

INTRODUCTION

The effects of fish oils in the diet have been studied extensively, and evidence is accumulating that eicosapentaenoic acid (EPA) and other polyunsaturated fatty acids may have a therapeutic effect on the cardiovascular system (1-3) (although not all researchers are in agreement on the effects). The National Institutes of Health have undertaken a program of clinical studies to determine the effects of fish oils on reducing cardiovascular infarction, and large amounts of EPA [and docosahexaenoic acid (DHA)] are being required for the clinical studies (4).

The clinical studies, in order to provide unequivocal results, require the fatty acids in a high degree of purity. Several methods can concentrate free fatty acids to high levels (i.e., 90+%). These include high-performance liquid chromatography (5), silver resin chromatography (6), urea crystallization (7), vacuum distillation

(8,9), and supercritical fluid fractionation (9-12). Some of these methods are excellent for analytical purposes at the laboratory level and some can be scaled up to production levels. Because EPA is heat-labile, the process of molecular distillation, commonly used in the purification of very low vapor pressure materials, is limited in its application to EPA concentration because of the high temperatures required to generate a reasonable separation factor. The advantages of supercritical fluid fractionation have been described in more detail previously (11,12). The results of the laboratory studies are extended to a continuous production process which can produce EPA in 90+% concentration (13).

PRINCIPLES OF SUPERCRITICAL FLUID FRACTIONATION OF FISH OILS

This chapter presents the advantages of supercritical fluid extraction for concentrating EPA and gives results of laboratory studies [taken primarily from two of the references (11,12)].

Supercritical fluid fractionation of fish oils is based on principles first reported over 100 years ago (14), viz., that many gases and liquids at condition above their critical points are solvents exhibiting pressure-dependent dissolving powers. An example of the pressure-dependent dissolving power of a supercritical fluid is given in Figure 1, which shows the solubility of naphthalene in carbon dioxide at 45°C. (The critical temperature of carbon dioxide is 31°C, the critical pressure 71 atm.) At low pressure (i.e., less than 50 atm), the solubility of naphthalene is seen to be very low, but as the critical pressure is increasingly exceeded the solubility rises to quite high levels, e.g., to 8-10% at 200 atm.

If carbon dioxide is considered to be "just a gas," solubility values of 8-10% might seem surprisingly high; carbon dioxide is not "just a gas," however. It exhibits a quite high density, about 0.85 g/cc at 45°C, 200 atm, for example, and the 0.85 g/cc density value is similar to that of many common laboratory and industrial solvents; thus, it is not unexpected that carbon dioxide might have a high dissolving power.

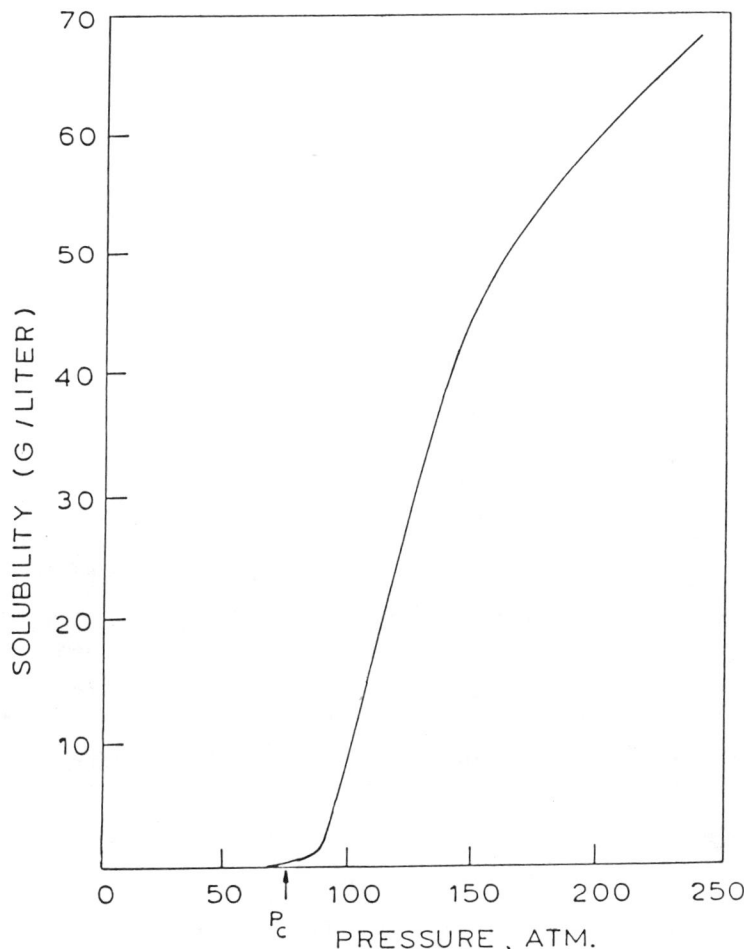

Figure 1 Solubility of naphthalene in carbon dioxide (45° C).

The advantageous thermodynamic and transport properties of supercritical fluids have been covered in many papers, books, and symposia proceedings (e.g., 15-19). It is adequate for present purposes to relate that the solubility behavior shown in Figure 1 is quite general for compounds soluble in supercritical fluids although the maximum concentration level of any compound in any gas under any set of conditions can be lower or higher than that shown in Figure 1. The same general behavior is shown by triglycerides in animal and vegetable oils; furthermore, in a mixture of homologous series triglycerides, components of different molecular weight will dissolve in a supercritical fluid to differentiate extents. For example, tributyrate and tricaproate will dissolve to a much greater extent than tristearate. This difference in solubility with molecular weight is not useful for the concentration of individual fatty acids from fish oils, however, because the fatty acid moieties are randomly positioned on the glycerol backbone. It is not at all likely that three EPA groups would be situated on one glycerol that could be extracted selectively by a supercritical fluid.

A compositional analysis of the fatty acids comprising menhaden oil which has been used as a feedstock for the preparation of high concentration EPA is given in Table 1; EPA content of this particular fish oil is about 16%. As already mentioned, supercritical fluid fractionation of fish oil (in triglyceride form) cannot concentrate the EPA, but if the triglycerides are saponified, and the fatty acid salts esterified to methyl or ethyl esters, the esters can be processed by supercritical fluid fractionation to achieve substantial concentration of EPA. As for the tributyrate-tristearate comparison given earlier, the C_{14}s will dissolve to a higher extent in supercritical carbon dioxide than will the C_{16}s or the C_{18}s, etc.

By appropriate manipulation of pressure (and temperature) supercritical fluid fractionation can, then, separate the mixture of esters by carbon number, i.e., the C_{18}s in a group, the C_{20}s in a group, etc. The maximum achievable concentration of EPA in the C_{20} fraction is calculable from material balance considerations, i.e., the ratio of EPA content to the content of total C_{20} fatty acids. Using menhaden ethyl esters, the "whole" esters in Table 1,

Table 1 Fatty Acid Profiles of the Whole Ester and Urea-Crystallized Ester Feedstocks

Fatty acid	Whole esters (%)	Urea crystallized esters (%)
14:0	7.8	—
16:0	15.6	—
16:1ω7	10.9	0.1
16:3ω4	1.1	5.3
16:4ω1	1.5	5.8
18:0	3.1	—
18:1ω9	7.6	—
18:1ω7	3.1	0.1
18:2ω6	1.3	0.2
18:3ω3	1.6	0.3
18:4ω3	2.9	7.6
20:1ω9	1.2	—
20:4ω6	1.0	1.4
20:4ω3	1.5	0.2
20:5ω3	16.5	48.6
22:5ω3	2.5	0.9
22:6ω3	10.9	22.2

Nilsson et al. achieved an EPA concentration close to the theoretically possible 72% using supercritical carbon dioxide (11). (Although any other of the common gases, such as methane, ethane, ethylene, etc., can be used to carry out the concentration of EPA, carbon dioxide is preferred because of its obvious safety and health and environmental attributes.)

In order to achieve a further enhancement in EPA concentration, for example, to values above 90%, which is desired for clinical trials, some of the unwanted C_{20} fatty esters must be removed by some other process. The process of urea crystallization allows separation to be made on the basis of fatty acid saturation; urea complexes preferentially with saturated and monounsaturated fatty acids and the solid complexes can be removed from the mixture, resulting in an enhanced concentration of polyunsaturated

components (7). Table 1 gives the composition of the esters resulting from the urea recystallization of ethyl esters of menhaden
oil. By removal of the saturated and monounsaturated esters the
EPA content has been increased from 15.8% to 48.6%, and a cal-
culation shows that a 97% EPA concentration fraction is theoretically possible using this feedstock; Nilsson et al. achieved a concentration of 96% (11), an excellent demonstration of the capabilities of supercritical fluid fractionation.

The technical capabilities of supercritical fluid fractionation
to produce very high concentration of EPA have been established
at the laboratory level, and the National Marine Fisheries Service
commissioned a study to determine the capital and operating costs
of a small pilot plant producing 10 lb/day of highly concentrated
(90+%) EPA at high yield (13). The study was also directed to the
design of a process more amenable to scaleup than the batch operation.

Figure 2 is a process flow diagram of a continuous countercurrent supercritical fluid concentration process. The flow diagram of Fig. 2 is similar to that of a high-pressure distillation process commonly used in the petroleum and petrochemicals industries. In brief description of the operation, a feed of urea-crystallized ethyl esters of fish oil is pumped into an extractor (Column
C-1). Based on a preliminary optimization using the data of Nilsson et al. (11), conditions of operation are chosen to be 60°C,
2200 psi. Carbon dioxide at these conditions is supplied to the
bottom of the extractor. As the carbon dioxide passes upward
through the downward-flowing esters, it extracts the more soluble
components from the ester stream, viz., the C_{14}s, C_{16}s, etc. The
resulting ester stream depleted in C_{14}s, C_{16}s, and C_{18}s leaves at the
bottom and is pumped to the second extractor (C-2). The carbon
dioxide stream laden with the light esters exists at the top of C-1
and is reduced in pressure slightly and raised in temperature; this
change in conditions causes the esters to "condense." Part of the
ester stream is returned to the extractor as "reflux," and part is
conveyed elsewhere. (The stream leaving the separator is termed
"light" in Fig. 2; it can be used for some other process or product,
or it can be discarded.) The carbon dioxide leaving the separator,

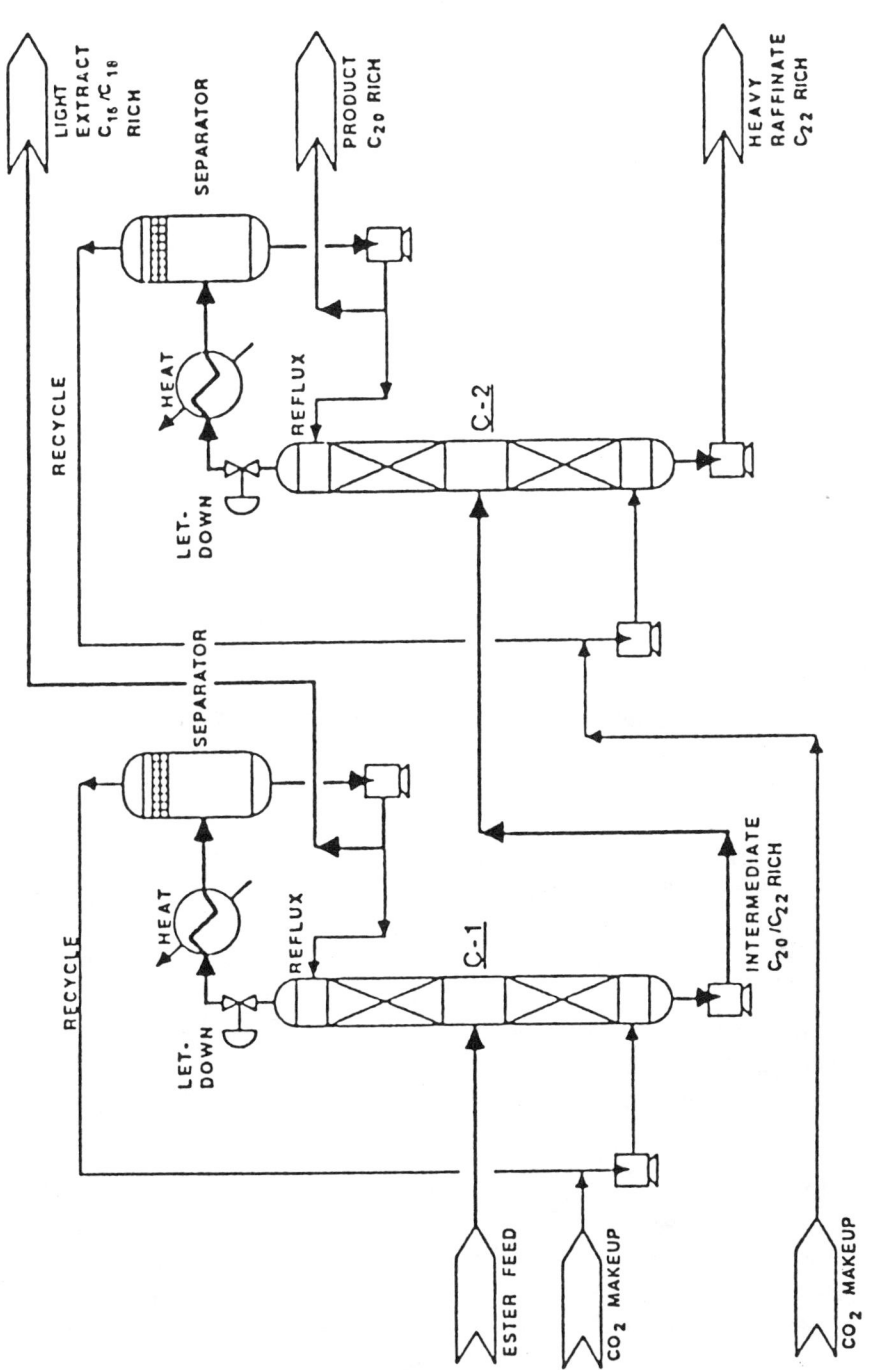

Figure 2 Process Flow Diagram--Supercritical Fluid Fractionation of Ethyl Esters of Fish Oil

and now essentially free of dissolved esters, is adjusted in temperature and pressure and returned to the bottom of the extractor, C-1. The "intermediate" stream leaving at the bottom of C-1 contains the C_{20}s and C_{22}s. This stream is pumped to Column C-2 and is separated into a C_{20}s stream and a C_{22}s stream. Operation of the second column is essentially identical to that in C-1. Based on the urea-crystallized ester feedstock with the composition shown in Table 1, a product stream is produced with a concentration of EPA of 90% or greater; simultaneously a stream with a docosahexaenic acid content of 90+% is produced.

The cost for producing a 90% EPA product in a small pilot plant operating at 10 lb/day has been estimated to be about $100/lb exclusive of the feed material costs. (The development of the capital and operating costs is covered in detail in Ref. 13.)

CLOSING REMARKS

Supercritical fluid extraction is being used commercially to decaffeinate coffee and to extract hops at levels of tens of millions of pounds per year, and thus, it is no longer the laboratory curiosity of 10 years ago.

Laboratory studies have shown that supercritical fluid fractionation is capable of separating the ethyl esters of fish oils to produce a product containing 90% EPA, and a preliminary design study has shown that the laboratory data can be scaled to large-volume production.

If, in the future, a product containing 90+% EPA is required at large volume, it is unlikely that any other process can produce it at less cost than supercritical fluid fractionation.

ACKNOWLEDGMENTS

The work of many people made this chapter possible. The experimental results of Dr. W. B. Nilsson have been used profusely. Mr. Charles J. Bambera, of Glitsch/Package Plants Div., carried out the process flow sheet and economics development, and Dr. J. E. Vivian, professor emeritus, Massachusetts Institute of Technology, carried out the conceptual column design. The funding from Mr. Roy E. Martin of the National Fish Meal and Oil Association under a Saltonstall-Kennedy Cooperative Agreement, NA-84AA-H-SK096, is gratefully acknowledged.

REFERENCES

1. Kromhout JM, Bossheiter EB, Coulander C. N Engl J Med 1985;312:1205.

2. Kremer JM, Michalek AVO, Lininger L, Huryck C, Bigarroette J. Lancet 1985;1:184.

3. Lands WEM. Fish and human health. Orlando, FL: Academic Press, 1986.

4. Nilsson WB. National Marine Fisheries Service, personal communication, 1988.

5. Aveldano MI, Van Rollins M, Harrocks LA. J Lipid Res 1983; 24:83.

6. Adlov RO, Emken EA. J Am Oil Chem Soc 1985;65:1592.

7. Sumerwell WN. J Am Chem Soc 1957;79:3411.

8. Ackman RG, Ke PJ, Jangaard PM. J Am Oil Chem Soc 1973; 50;1.

9. Eisenbach W. Ber Bunsenges Phys Chem 1984;88:882.

10. Krukonis VJ. Supercritical fluid fractionation of fish oils: concentration of eicosapentaenoic acid, presented at 75th Ann. Americal Oil Chemical Society meeting, Dallas, April 1984.

11. Nilsson WB, Gauglitz EJ Jr, Hudson JK, Stout VF, Spinelli J. J Am Oil Chem Soc 1988;65:109.

12. Krukonis VJ. Continuous process for the production of high concentration EPA, presented at American Chemical Society meeting, New Orleans, September 1987.

13. Krukonis VJ. Design of a continuous counter-current fractionation process for producing concentrated EPA ethyl es-

ters, Appendix A to Final Report submitted to National Fish Meal and Oil Association, Washington, DC.

14. Hannary JB, Hogarth J. Proc Roy Soc London 1879;29:324.

15. McHugh MA, Krukonis VJ. Supercritical fluid extraction: principles and practice. Stoneham, MA: Butterworth, 1986.

16. Penninger JML, Radosz M, McHugh MA, Krukonis VJ, eds. Supercritical fluid technology, Process Technology Proceedings, 3. Amsterdam: Elsevier, 1985.

17. Squires TG, Paulaitis ME, eds. Supercritical fluids: chemical and engineering principles and applications, ACS Symposium Series #329. American Chemical Society, Washington, DC, 1987.

18. Stahl E, Quirin KW, Gerard D. High pressure gases for extraction and refining. Berlin: Springer Verlag, 1987.

19. Charpentier BA, Sevanants MR, eds. Supercritical fluid extraction and chromatography: techniques and applications, ACS Symposium Series #366. American Chemical Society, Washington, DC, 1988.

9
Omega-3 Fatty Acids from Algae

Richard J. Radmer
Martek Corporation
Columbia, Maryland

INTRODUCTION

In this chapter, I briefly describe an interesting and potentially valuable source of omega-3 fatty acids, the marine microalgae.

Many species of algae are known to produce significant quantities of the omega-3 fatty acids, eicosapentaenoic acid (EPA) and docosahexaenoic acid (DHA). In fact, according to some investigators, much or all of these compounds contained in fish originate in algae and work their way up through the food chain. It is not my intent to prove or disprove this view. What I do intend to do is point out some of the unique qualities of microalgal sources of EPA and DHA and to illustrate their potential advantages in research, medical, and commercial applications.

The relative abundance of specific fatty acids, in particular the polyunsaturated fatty acids (PUFAs), can be considered a fingerprint of a particular species of marine microalga. For example, species in the class Bacillariophyceae (diatoms) contain large

211

Table 1 Profiles of Several Omega-3 Fatty Acid Sources (%)

Fatty acid	Commercial oils		Fish fillets		Microlage	
	Cod liver	MaxEPA	Bluefish	Salmon	MK-8600	MK-8620
14.0	5.5	4.6	5.7	9.4	4.1	2.9
14.1	1.4	1.3	<1	<1	<1	<1
16.0	7.7	6.4	19	12	21.1	9.9
16.1	10.1	7.0	8.8	7.9	48	60
16.2	1.4	2.4	<1	<1	2.0	2.3
18.0	2.5	3.3	9.5	4.2	<1	<1
18.1	16.5	9.9	22	20	2.8	2.3
18.2	2.8	3.8	1.8	3.1	2.2	<1
18.3	<1	<1	<1	<1	5.7	<1
20.1	14.5	7.7	5.1	8.3	1.1	<1
20.5 EPA	9.9	15.1	3.4	4.6	11	21
22.1	10.9	7.2	4.3	8.2	<1	<1
22.6 DHA	10.2	13.2	14	7.7	2.0	<1
Extractable oil in biomass (%)	—	—	3.9	19	51	28
EPA in dry biomass (%)	—	—	0.1	0.9	5.6	5.9

amounts of EPA and little DHA, whereas those in the Dinophyceae (dinoflagellates) have predominantly DHA (e.g., Ref. 1,2). Table 1 summarizes the fatty acid profiles of cod liver oil, MaxEPA (a commercially available omega-3 PUFA preparation), two species of fish, and two algal strains from the Martek culture collection. Note that the omega-3 abundance in the lipid of these algae is at least as high as in the fish preparations, and that there is a complete absence of DHA in one of the algal strains. Furthermore, these algal strains contain large oil droplets and have a much higher net oil content than oily fish such as salmon. Consequently, the algae have an EPA content at least 10-fold higher than the fish on a dry weight basis (Table 1). Indeed, since many of these same algal species produce lipids as a storage product, they can be considered natural overproducers of omega-3 PUFAs.

In addition to the production of large amounts of PUFAs, the use of these organisms in culture offers distinct advantages over dependence on harvested wild populations such as fish. Microalgae provide great potential for enhancing the productivity of components of interest through genetic modification and strain selection, using approaches that have been so successful in enhancing antibiotic production by microorganisms in culture. Recently, a research effort at Martek led by Dr. David Kyle, under the auspices of the National Institutes of Health, has established several species of EPA-producing organisms (primarily diatoms) in axenic culture. Subsequent studies demonstrated that proper control of culture conditions resulted in a 10-fold increase in the relative EPA content of these organisms. Dr. Kyle and his colleagues have also developed techniques for the preparation and purification of algal oil and/or pure EPA from these organisms. Several of these EPA-producing lines have subsequently been grown under heterotrophic conditions, which could provide the opportunity to produce the algal EPA using conventional fermentation equipment and procedures.

An interesting preliminary observation from this work was that the EPA in algal oil exhibited a greater degree of oxidative stability than that in fish oil. The nature of the stabilizing agent in the algal oil is unknown, but the unexpected benefit is that an EPA-containing algal oil undergoes very little PUFA oxidation and has no apparent "fishy" odor or taste.

The future use of EPA (or oils containing EPA) for treatment of various disorders will require extensive clinical trials. This, in turn, will require large quantities of EPA-containing oil with a standard composition, delivered on a regular, reliable basis. These algal-based processes could provide a reliable, economically attractive EPA source for the research and clinical trials. These organisms also provide the means to produce other related products, such as EPA labeled with deuterium, ^{13}C, or ^{14}C, and genes that code for EPA production. In addition to these direct clinical and pharmaceutical applications, algae provide a means to develop a source of EPA-containing oil compatible with foods in the normal human diet. This latter possibility is likely to have the greatest influence on the health of the average person, since it does not require the purchase of pills or the recognition and treatment of a clinical disorder. Rather, it could represent a preventive medicine available to, and supplied to, the general public, analogous to fluoridated water or vitamin-supplemented foods. These are clearly lofty goals, and a good deal of additional investigation is required to establish whether or not such an application has a legitimate clinical basis.

REFERENCES

1.   Cohen Z. In: Richmond A, ed. Handbook of microalgal mass culture. Boca Raton, FL: CRC Press, 1986: 421-454.

2.   Loeblich AR, Loeblich LA. In: Laskin AL, Lechevalier HA, eds. CRC handbook of microbiology, Vol. II, 2nd ed. West Palm Beach, FL: CRC Press, 1978: 425-250.

10
Chemical and Analytical Aspects of Assuring an Effective Supply of Omega-3 Fatty Acids to the Consumer

Robert G. Ackman and W. M. N. Ratnayake*
Canadian Institute of Fisheries Technology
Technical University of Nova Scotia
Halifax, Nova Scotia, Canada

FISH OR FISH OILS AS SOURCES OF OMEGA-3 FATTY ACIDS

Promoters of increased fish and shellfish in the diet can argue that fish oils or lipids act as "carriers" for a variety of chemicals concentrated from the environment, as well as biogenic materials about which we often know so little. Promoters of fish oils as omega-3 sources can argue that shellfish carry certain diseases and that fish oils made from reduction of whole fish might be unwholesome. Additionally, one can argue that some fatty fish have low contents of omega-3 fatty acids, adding unnecessarily to calories, or that severe processing and refining conditions for fish oils would create artifacts with unknown biochemical effects.

Fatty Acids of Fish Oils

Fish oils are not as complex a problem as they once appeared. For this brief review, shark liver oils (including Atlantic and Pacific

---

* Food Directorate, Health and Welfare Canada, Ottawa, Ontario, Canada

215

dogfish oils) and toothed whale oils will be omitted as they often contain glyceryl ethers, wax esters, or hydrocarbons such as pristane or squalene, which make them unsuitable as sources of omega-3 acids. This leaves as much as 1 million tons of commercial fish oils available in triglyceride form (usually about 98% triglyceride).

There are eight fatty acids of most interest in marine oils. In a shorthand notation of chain length and number of double bonds these are:

			Iodine value (IV)
Saturated	Myristic acid	14:0	NIL
	Palmitic acid	16:0	NIL
Monounsaturated	Palmitoleic acid	16:1	100
	Oleic acid	18:1	90
	Gadoleic acid	20:1	82
	Cetoleic acid	22:1	75
Polyunsaturated	Eicosapentaenoic acid	20:5n-3 (or EPA)	420
	Docosahexaenoic acid	22:6n-3 (or DHA)	464

In marine fish oils the "omega-6" fatty acids are usually 1-2% of the total, but only one of interest, arachidonic acid (20:4n-6), will concentrate along with EPA in most enrichment technology. It is usually 1/10th to 1/20th of the EPA present. Minor polyunsaturated C_{20} and C_{22} omega-3 fatty acids may also be enriched by some methods.

Freshwater fish oils have C_{20} omega-6 fatty acids with totals roughly equal to omega-3 content, and this would be true of fish lipids and oils from most tropical and some semitropical fish (e.g., Northern Australia). On the other hand, cold-water sea fish from Tasmania, New Zealand, South Africa, Argentina, and Chile resemble North Atlantic and North Pacific fish oils in fatty acid composition.

Commercially available oils have iodine values ranging from about 95 (certain Atlantic herring oils) to 195 (pilchard oils). As

an example, an Atlantic menhaden oil of IV 167 has 27.5% polyunsaturated C_{18}, C_{20}, and C_{22} acids of biochemical or commercial
interest, plus 3-4% of C_{16} polyunsaturated acids, which are often
not tabulated as they are not recognized by some analysts. It is
important to emphasize that EPA + DHA usually total about 80%
of all polyunsaturated fatty acids in marine oils.

The fish body oils (Table 1) may be divided into two groups,
those with 14% or more of 20:1-22:1 fatty acids and those with
less. This reflects feeding patterns, as the 20:1 and 22:1 are of
dietary origin (Ackman et al., 1980). If a fish (for example, Atlantic herring) feeds heavily on certain small crustacea, it will convert

Table 1   Some Major Marine Oils of Commerce, with Approximate Iodine Values, Weight Percentages of Saturated Acids, 20:1 +
22:1, and EPA + DHA

Oil	IV	Sat. (%)	20:1 + 22:1 (%)	EPA + DHA (%)
Body oils				
Herring (Atlantic)	125	19	35	14
Capelin	125	18	36	11
Redfish	125	21	36	9
Herring (Pacific)	140	34	10	7
Sand launce	140	24	27	17
Mackerel	150	27	38	15
Salmon (Pacific)	150	26	17	19
Sardine	160	30	8	24
Menhaden	162	32	2	20
Anchovy	181	30	3	26
Pilchard	185	28	5	26
Liver oils				
Cod (Atlantic)	165	21	13	24
Pollock (Alaska)	160	18	30	17
Squid (Pacific)	180	21	17	28
Other				
Salmon egg (Pacific)	210	?	?	?
Seal (Atlantic)	150	14	17	14

long-chain (20:1 and 22:1) alcohols from the crustacea into fatty acids and put them into the 3 position on the fish triglycerides. Synthesis of the triglycerides is necessary for the animal to lay down depot fat reserves, and there is a tendency for dietary polyunsaturated fatty acids to be inserted via a phospholipid in the 2 position. The fish is free to deposit dietary fatty acids such as 14:0, 16:0, 16:1, or 18:1 or to biosynthesize any of these to fill in the 1 position. If no 20:1 or 22:1 is provided by the diet, then it will put any available fatty acids into the 3 position. The anomalous result is that, in general, the higher the iodine value of a fish body oil, the higher the total saturated acids. Note the difference in saturated acids between Atlantic and Pacific herring oils in Table 1 relative to 20:1 + 22:1.

The result of these two different types of fish body oils being available is that if there is little or no 20:1 + 22:1, then EPA and DHA are usually high, perhaps 20% of total fatty acids. If much 20:1 and 22:1 are present, then they dilute the EPA and DHA down to as little as 8-10% total.

No mention has been made of 16:1 and 18:1 in Table 1. These two fatty acids seem to be to some extent interchangeable; for example, their totals are the same in sand launce oils from the North Sea and from off Nova Scotia, although the proportions differ. Similarly 14:0 and 16:0 may be interchangeable, although 16:0 is always the most important.

Although there is no known specific reason for the observation, the maximum for polyunsaturated fatty acids in marine oil triglycerides seems to be about 1 mole, putting a finite limit on concentration of omega-3 acids as natural triglycerides. The triglycerides examined to date always represent a group with similar chromatographic or physical properties. There are, therefore, hundreds of types of molecules in any marine oil or fraction, no matter how the latter is isolated. Moreover, the values given in Table 1 are typical for one lot of oil. Herring oils, for example, can have IVs as low as 95 and as high as 150. Menhaden oils have IVs ranging at times as low as 145 in the Gulf of Mexico fishery. The fish liver oils usually have 22:1 $\geqslant$ 20:1, and 20:5 $\approx$ 22:6, so they should be considered separately. It appears that for practical purposes there is only *one* marine fish body oil (i.e., menhaden or pilchard type), with properties modified by extra 20:1 and 22:1 (Ackman et al., 1987).

Nontriglyceride Components

It is not generally realized that fish oils contain about 0.5% of dissolved water. It is often associated with polar impurities, but will be found even in refined oils unless they are vacuum-stripped at high temperature.

All fish oils contain 0.5-1.0% sterol, usually more than 95% cholesterol. There are commercial oils which can contain up to 2% wax esters, and some contain free alcohols, often mostly hexadecanol CH_3-$(CH_2)_{14}$-CH_2OH, but at times including 20:1 and 22:1 alcohols (Ratnayake and Ackman, 1979). Much depends on whether the oils are from reduction of feeding fish, with stomach contents included, or from fish muscle scrap, but there are in any case strong seasonal variations.

The hydrocarbon pristane may be up to 0.1% of fish oils, again with strong seasonal variations. Other hydrocarbons are relatively minor and usually aliphatic (e.g., heptadecane). Formerly whale oil produced in factory ships was put into empty fuel tanks, so tests for fuel oil in whale oil were part of the industry. This is not anticipated as a problem with contemporary fish oils, but accidents do happen.

Tocopherol, exclusively as the alpha isomer, will be about 300 $\mu g/g$ of raw fish oils. Together with the carotenoid pigments found in some lots of fish oils, it will have chemical antioxidant properties, but if eliminated it is easily put back into products as a "biochemical" antioxidant.

PCBs are found at 2-5 ppm in almost all fish oils (Addison and Ackman, 1974). They are not affected by any refining step except vacuum deodorization (Addison et al., 1978), which effectively removes PCBs to less than detectable levels. In the margarine industry deodorization was a posthydrogenation process carried out under quite severe conditions of temperature (250°C) and vacuum (2-5 mm Hg). Milder conditions executed to clean up

the off-flavors of natural cod liver oils also seem to be quite effective. The DDT products, such as DDE, should be equally well
eliminated. Phthalates occur in all fish oils and are easily added
in laboratory handling. They are less likely to be a problem in
large-scale handling of oils.

Our experience in Halifax with a Pope 6-in., wiped-wall still,
run under vacuum as a stripper, is that PCBs are readily removed
from fish oils at moderate (ca. 200°C) temperatures, eliminating
risk of thermal hazard to EPA and DHA. The throughput could
be as high as 30-50 kg/h, and this unit, the largest from the Pope
company, runs continuously with little or no attention. Tests are
continuing.

Free fatty acids at 1-3% of oil weight are common in fish
oils. These are titrated and reported as w/w% oleic acid (18:1)
but in fact can be any of the fish fatty acids present in the oil.
If the oil is badly oxidized, some of the volatile fatty acids (C_2 -
C_6) can be present, but this oil would not usually be acceptable
for any high-quality use. Refining by established techniques
(Addison et al., 1978) reduces these to about 0.1%. Preliminary
results from the Pope unit described above suggest that it is also
effective in removing free fatty acids.

Mono- and diglycerides are present but are seldom reported
as levels are very low in all oils, except in "cod" oil from autolysed
livers. They mostly reflect the enzyme activity during holding of
the fish prior to reduction, rather than being from chemical hydrolysis.

Heavy metals are natural trace components in *all* edible oils,
of either plant or fish origin. Regulations such as that of FAO
include limits of 0.1 μg/g for copper, lead, and arsenic. Of these
arsenic is probably present in association with phospholipids and
is dramatically reduced by conventional oil refining from as much
as 10 μg/g in crude oils to <0.1 μg/g. Data are available for Cu,
Cd, Pb, As, Zn, Hg, and Se (Elson and Ackman, 1978; Elson et al.,
1981; see Tables 2 and 3). Some of these elements are believed to
be included in actual fatty acids rather than in unsaponifiable
matter. If so, they may not concentrate in any oil fraction but
could be enriched in concentrates of fatty acids or esters.

Table 2 The Metal Content of Herring Oil at Various Processing ($\mu g/g$) and Comparable Data

Oil stage	Metal						
	Hg	Se	As	Zn	Cd	Pb	Cu
Original data[a]							
Lot 1 crude	0.010 ± 0.009	0.047 ± 0.008	4.0 ± 0.2	5.1 ± 1.4	0.007 ± 0.001	0.13 ± 0.01	0.21 ± 0.03
Lot 1 bleached		0.041 ± 0.005	<0.1	3.4 ± 1.2	0.001 ± 0.001	0.11 ± 0.02	0.10 ± 0.02
Lot 1 partially hydrogenated (Ni) and deodorized	0.004 ± 0.008	<0.003	<0.1	6.6 ± 1.2	0.004 ± 0.001	0.08 ± 0.01	0.19 ± 0.03
Lot 2 partially hydrogenated (Ni) and deodorized	—	—	—	—	0.001 ± 0.001	0.08 ± 0.01	<0.05
Literature data							
Crude marine[b] oil	—	—	8-14	—	—	—	—
Hydrogenated marine oil	—	—	<0.2	—	—	—	0.004 ± 0.04
Refined fish oil	<0.01	—	0.02	—	0.008	0.08	—
Crude herring oil	—	0.02-0.09	5.3-6.5	—	—	—	—
Hydrogenated herring oil	<0.02	—	—	—	—	—	—
Crude fish press oil	0.34	—	0.16	—	0.004	0.05	—

[a]Elson and Ackman (1978).
[b]Marine = herring, mackerel, capelin.

Table 3 The Metal Content of Menhaden Oil at Different Stages of Processing ($\mu g/g$)[a]

Oil stage	Metal				
	Cd	Pb	Cu	As	Zn
Crude	0.04 ± 0.01	0.32 ± 0.05	0.23 ± 0.003	10.4 ± 0.7	64.9 ± 13.3
Degummed	0.04 ± 0.01	0.08 ± 0.04	0.10 ± 0.004	1.8 ± 0.1	8.3 ± 1.1
Degummed plus gums	0.02 ± 0.01	0.06 ± 0.02	0.13 ± 0.02	2.0 ± 0.9	9.0 ± 1.1
Refined	0.02 ± 0.01	0.09 ± 0.03	0.08 ± 0.04	Bdl[b]	2.7 ± 0.4
Refined and bleached	0 01 ± 0.00	0.04 ± 0.03	0.04 ± 0.03	Bdl	Bdl
Hydrogenated (Ni) and filtered	0.02 ± 0.01	0.03 ± 0.00	0.04 ± 0.01	Bdl	Bdl
Hydrogenated, filtered, and bleached	Bdl	0.06 ± 0.02	0.04 ± 0.01	Bdl	Bdl
Hydrogenated, filtered, bleached, and deodorized	Bdl	0.05 ± 0.02	0.06 ± 0.01	Bdl	Bdl

[a]Elson et al. (1981).
[b]Bdl = below detection limit of wet digestion and as measurement (0.005 $\mu g/g$ Cd; 0.7 $\mu g/g$ As; 0.8 $\mu g/g$ Zn; 0.02 $\mu g/g$ Pb).

The oxidation of fish oils is inevitable. In a large tank free oxygen can be measured down to a depth of a few centimeters; then it is no longer present. In some oils sulfur and nitrogen compounds from muscle contribute to the "fishy flavor." The "rancidity" flavor of all fish oils includes a variety of aldehydes, often unsaturated, of which 2-*trans*, 4-*cis*, 7-*cis*-decatrienal is considered especially important as a specific product of EPA and DHA. The other oxidation products may be found in most meats and in vegetable oils. In a mackerel oil of peroxide value 15, alkanals (in moles/g $\times 10^{-9}$) totaled 73, alkenols 1.6, alkadienals 0.3, and the decatrienal <0.1 (Ke et al., 1975). TBHQ is the best chemical antioxidant for fish oils, ethoxyquin is next, and BHA/BHT the next most efficient.

OIL FRACTIONATION

Winterization of Triglycerides

The higher content of saturated fatty acids in the fish body oils of higher IV (Table 1) has an important consequence. Such oils can usually be "winterized" by slow cooling to about 5°C. There are also data for menhaden oil (Ackman, 1981):

	Starting oil	Stearine	Winterized liquid layer
IV	175	136	187
w/w% saturated	35.7	49.3	32.1
w/w% mononunsaturated	27.1	22.4	27.2
w/w% polyunsaturated	37.2	28.3	40.7
w/w% EPA + DHA	23.6	23.1	33.3

The vital observation is that two quite different classes of molecules are involved. Since the menhaden stearine, and presumably most other fish oil stearines, contain over 20% EPA + DHA, the difference may reflect two saturated acids per molecule in many of the stearine triglycerides. By assuming that the saturated acids are 16:0, monounsaturated acids are 18:1, and polyunsaturated acids are EPA, the weight percents for the menhaden oil stearine can be converted to mole%:

$$49.3 \div 254 = 0.194 = 53 \text{ mole}\% \text{ (saturated)}$$
$$22.4 \div 282 = 0.079 = 22 \text{ mole}\% \text{ (monounsaturated)}$$
$$28.3 \div 302 = \underline{0.094} = 25 \text{ mole}\% \text{ (polyunsaturated)}$$
$$0.367$$

This approximation is satisfactorily close as evidence that stearine is partly a defined chemical class of disaturated triglyceride and that the other fatty acids in such triglycerides may be either mono- or polyunsaturated. Part of the stearine will be made up of molecules "fitting" into the basic crystals irrespective of fatty acid composition.

Molecular Distillation of Triglycerides and Thermal Hazard

The result of winterizing is to produce an oil with increased omega-3 content with no use of solvents. The only other technology capable of enrichment of oils without solvents is molecular distillation. This process requires very high vacuum, at least of the order of 10^{-6} mm Hg. It is a short-path process, typically with the distance from the evaporator to condensing surface being 1-3 cm. There is no provision of reflux, so the distillation efficiency generally is less than one plate and reflects molecular weight differences. As shown in Figure 1, a Japanese sardine oil does seem to have a group of triglycerides of low molecular weight not reported for any of the fish oils listed in Table 1. These can be presumed to have a low probability of containing EPA and DHA and their removal by molecular distillation should leave a greater proportion of EPA and DHA in the residue. With repeated passes of an oil low in 20:1 and 22:1, the residue will be progressively enriched in high-molecular-weight combinations.

In distilling individual fatty acid esters there is a problem with thermal hazard to the EPA and DHA. The pressure drop in an efficient packed column is such that pot temperatures of up to 250° may be required to obtain distillates boiling at 180° at 1-2

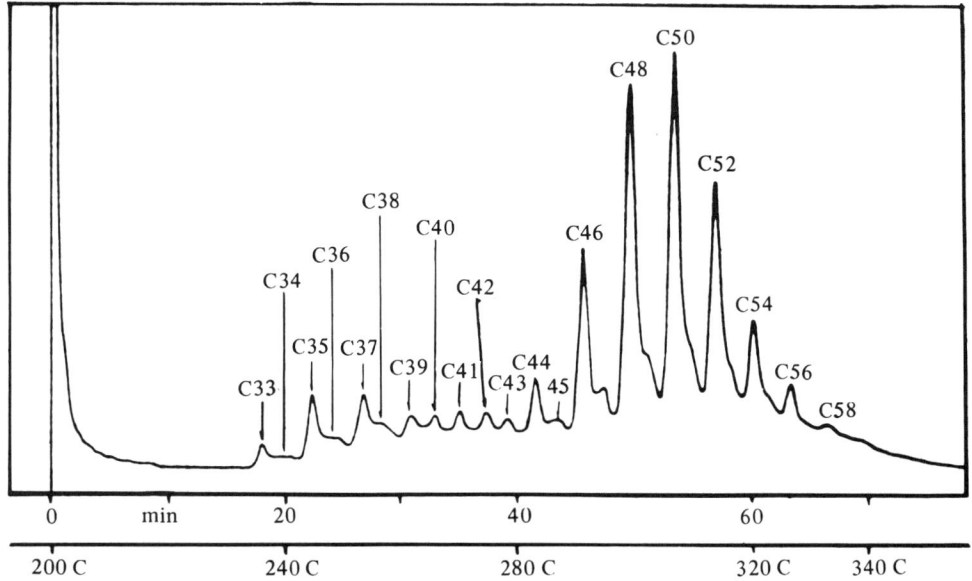

Figure 1   Gas-liquid chromatography of triglycerides of Japanese sardine oil. Note substantial proportion of unusual C_{33} -C_{43} triglycerides and maximum at C_{50}. From Ikekawa et al. (1972).

mm pressure. Figure 2 shows artifact development and destruction of EPA and DHA for such a distillation. Spinning band columns should have a lower pressure drop and still be efficient enough to remove C_{14} and C_{16} fatty acids as esters. In terms of the molecular weight, the loss of 10 hydrogens from 20:0 to give 20:5 (EPA) is almost the same as loss of one methylene carbon, so 20:5 will be similar in boiling point to a C_{19} fatty acid ester. This may hinder full removal of the C_{18} materials without loss of EPA.

Solvent Crystallization of Triglycerides

Solvent crystallization speeds up winterization, but has several problems despite numerous patents on the subject in the 1940s. Oils are inherently insoluble in solvents at low tempertures, although acetone is perhaps suitable, so solvent volumes are large.

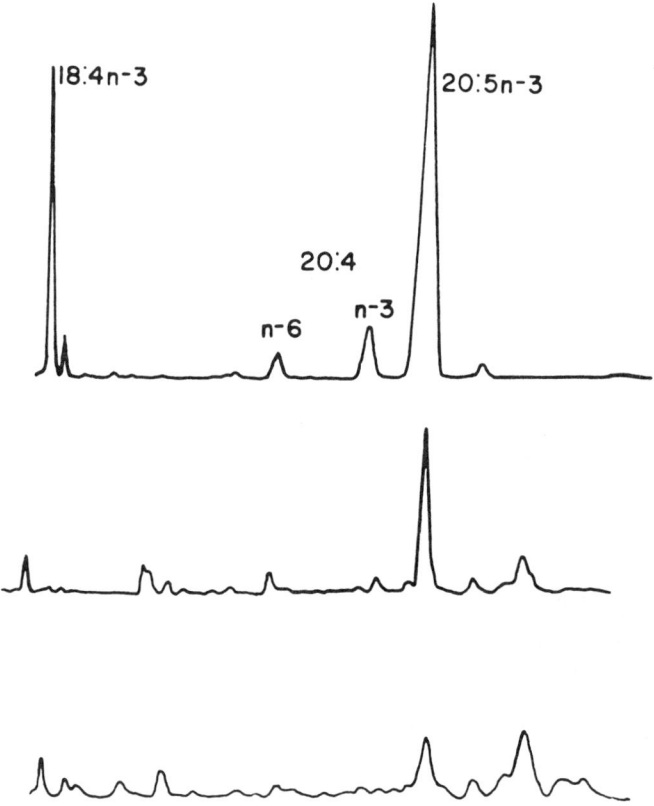

Figure 2 Gas-liquid chromatography showing artifacts produced during Stedmann column distillation of a concentrate of ethyl esters of fish oil fatty acids. Top, starting material; center, distillate; bottom, pot residue.

Directed Intesterification

In theory this commercial process, developed by Eckey for lard, tallow, margarine and shortenings, palm oil, etc., could be adapted for fish oils. By very slowly chilling a solution of oil in xylene or other solvent, and in the presence of an alkaline earth catalyst such as sodium alcoholate, newly formed higher-melting triglycerides should crystallize out. This could be useful for herring and similar oils with a high content of 20:1 and 22:1, but to date no reports have appeared on successful application of the technique to produce oils enriched in EPA and DHA. It is possible that the fatty acids of mixed chain lengths common in fish oils, randomized on the glycerol molecule, do not solidify readily. Most successful cases have involved a narrow range (C_{16} or C_{18}) of chain lengths amenable to crystal formation.

Other Oil Enrichment Techniques

Countercurrent column fractionation was tested in Halifax with a 1 in. $\times$ 6 ft Karr pulsed countercurrent column. The results were judged not economically practical with oil as the nonpolar phase. As resources did not permit a test with oil in solution or a thorough test of solvents and temperatures, this work is in abeyance. Generally, impurities tend to concentrate in the extract along with the desired triglycerides enriched in EPA and DHA.

Chromatography has been described in Japanese patients but all processes involve large volumes of solvents. The life of column packings is always problematical. Porous polymers plug up, silicic acid is slightly soluble in some solvents, and the acceptable load on reversed-phase packings is very low. If the rest of the fish oil can be salvaged, then in principle a small proportion (1-2%) of oil might be recoverable enriched in EPA or DHA.

Supercritical CO_2 separation reports are rare but appear to show that oils are *not* very satisfactory raw materials and that esters are preferred.

Esters and Acids

Nature has not been kind in assembling fish oil triglycerides, and logic therefore indicates that free acids and their esters are much more favorable points of attack in concentration processes since the three basic types of fatty acids can have radially different physical properties.

Saponification has the advantage (in theory) that *all* unsaponifiables can be removed and a clean fatty acid fraction made the process raw material. This would require one or more solvents in

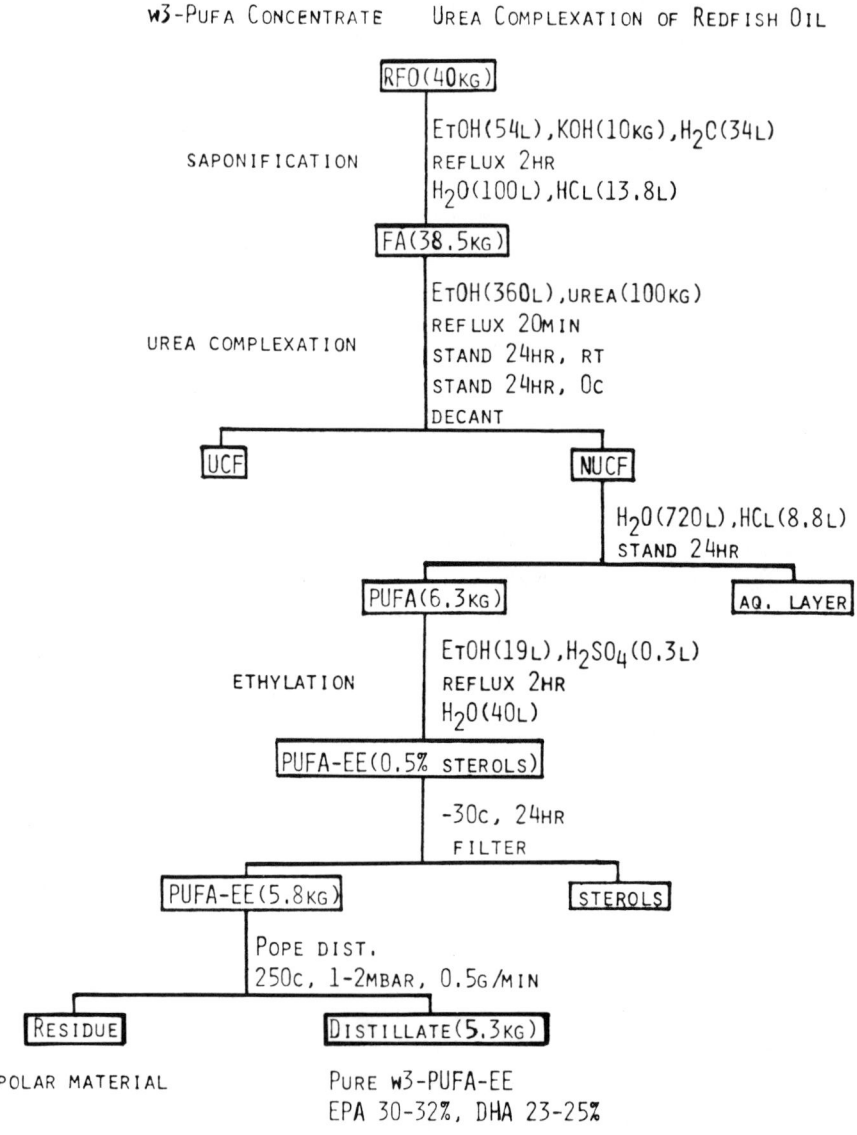

Figure 3 Flow process to enrich polyunsaturated fatty acids by urea complexation of saturated, and monounsaturated, fatty acids of commercial redfish (*Sebastes* spp.) oil. Distillation rate for NUCF esters refers to Pope 2-in. model.

some quantity (for example, hexane or methylene chloride) and probably a centrifuge separation. As the urea process flow sheet shows (Fig. 3) simple saponification in ethanol-water gives a clean free acid on gravity separation, with a trace of ethyl ester formation. Fat-soluble impurities are also enriched along with EPA and DHA if they do not form urea complexes, but if 80% of the fatty acids are readily eliminated then the expense for final cleanup (of the 20%) is much reduced.

Low-temperature crystallization of acids or esters is much simpler than for oils, and iodine values of concentrates rise by 50-100 units for fatty acids of menhaden oil for 50% yield of filtrate (Bailey, 1952). Fatty acids of a (Pacific) herring oil of IV 138 yielding 22% of a fraction of IV 297 from a 10% solution in petroleum ether at -70°C. The latter product should have been over 50% (EPA + DHA). Probably, free acids are better than esters for crystallization as they are more soluble.

Urea complexation (see Fig. 3 flow sheet) can be applied to either acids or esters. We have preferred to use acids, the U.S. National Marine Fisheries Service prefers ethyl esters, but in either case 70% omega-3 acids (50-60% of EPA + DHA) is readily obtained. The ratio of EPA to DHA is nearly the same as in the starting oil.

Chromatographic procedures are also more practical for acids or esters than they were for oils. Analytical high-performance liquid chromatography separations are very promising (Fig. 4). On the other hand, a column of 50 mm diameter, 5 mm in length, with several thousand dollars worth of reversed-phase packings, will accept only a few hundred milligrams of esters if the separation is to be at all efficient. At least several liters of solvent will be required, so it is clear that this process can only be used for final separations.

Solvents

The use of solvents creates a number of problems. Because fish oils contain EPA and DHA as well as other unsaturated fatty acids, there is inevitable oxidation. At one extreme, involatile gums,

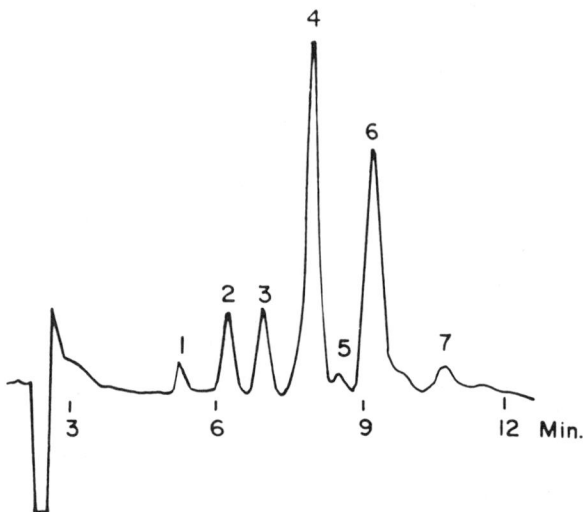

Figure 4 Analytical scale HPLC of concentrate of ethyl esters such as are produced by urea complexation of unwanted fatty acids (Fig. 3). Peak 4 contains 86% EPA, peak 6 92% DHA. C_{18} μ-Bondapak column, 25 cm $\times$ 4 mm, solvent MeOH: H_2O: 95:5.

varnishes, and polymers accumulate in equipment, and at the other, a host of volatile ($\leqslant C_{10}$) hydrocarbons, acids, aldehydes, ketones, esters, and peroxides accumulate in solvents. Past experience shows that some of these form azeotropes with solvents and hence are very difficult to remove even by efficient fractional distillation. A charcoal treatment step may be necessary if solvents are frequently recycled.

When fish oils or esters are manipulated, there is always darkening and a bleaching step may be necessary unless a final purification step is distillation, in which case the pigmentation usually stays in the residue. The Pope wiped wall still has a very short residence time and thermal hazard risk is negligible.

Table 4   Wt% Branched-Chain Fatty Acids in Omega-3 PUFA
Concentrates from Different Fish Oils

Fatty acid	Oil		
	Menhaden	Redfish	Salmon
Iso-14	TR	TR	TR
4,8,12-TMTD	0.2	0.2	0.3
11-MTD	TR	0.1	0.2
Iso-15	0.1	0.4	0.1
Aiso-15	0.1	0.3	0.1
5,9,13-TMTD[a]	TR	TR	TR
Iso-16	TR	0.1	0.1
2,6 10,14-TMPD	0.2	0.4	0.4
2,2,6,10,14-PMPD[a]	ND	0.5	ND
7-MHD	0.4	0.9	3.2
11-MHD[a]	TR	TR	0.1
13-MHD[a]	TR	TR	0.1
7,8-DMHD[a]	0.1	0.1	2.3
3,7,11,14-TMHD	0.9	0.6	0.4
2,3,7,11,15-PMHD[a]	ND	0.4	ND
Iso-18	TR	0.1	0.3

[a]Novel fatty acids not previously known in fish oils. TR = trace; M = methyl.
For details see Ratnayake et al., 1989.

Novel Fatty Acids in Concentrates

Our urea process is a natural first step to the examination of fish
oils for minor and possibly novel fatty acids. The degree of enrichment can be as high as fivefold. Table 4 shows the details for
minor saturated fatty acids of three fish oils as indicated by GC-
MS. The redfish oil provided two unusual fatty acids with novel 2-
methyl branched structures, related to the known pristanic (2,6,
10,14-tetramethylpentadecanoic) and phytanic (3,7,11,15-tetra-
methylhexadecanoic) acids. The others are mostly monomethyl
branched fatty acids and none are expected to be physiologically
important. More work is needed on the minor components of
fish oils, including non-fatty acid components. Despite the excellent health record of fish as food, there is enough difference in

Table 4 with respect to the 2-methyl branched isoprenoid acids to suggest that all fish oil sources and concentrates need further study.

ACKNOWLEDGMENT

The cooperation of Pope Scientific Inc., N90 W14337 Commerce Drive, Memomonee Falls, WI 53051-9990, is gratefully acknowledged. The research was supported in part by the Natural Sciences Research and Engineering Council of Canada.

REFERENCES

Ackman RG. Fish lipids. In: Connell JJ, ed. Advances in fish science and technology. Farnham, Surrey: Fishing News Books, 1981: 86-103.

Ackman RG, Sebedio JL, Kovacs MIP. Role of eicosenoic and docosenoic fatty acids in freshwater and marine lipids. Marine Chem 1980 9:157-164.

Ackman RG, Ratnayake WMN, Olsson B. The "basic" fatty acid composition of Atlantic fish oils: potential similarities useful for enrichment of polyunsaturated fatty acids by urea complexation. J Am Oil Chem Soc 1987;65:136-138.

Addison RF, Ackman RG. Removal of organochlorine pesticides and polychlorinated biphenyls from marine oils during refining and hydrogenation for edible use. J Am Oil Chem Soc 1974;51:192-194.

Addison RF, Zinck ME, Ackman RG, Sipos JC. Behavior of DDT, polychlorinated biphenyls (PCBs), and dieldrin at various stages of refining of marine oils for edible use. J Am Oil Chem Soc 1978;55:391-394.

Bailey RE, ed. Marine oils with particular reference to those of Canada. Bull. 89, Fisheries Research Board of Canada. Ottowa, 1952.

Elson CM, Ackman RG. Trace metal content of a herring oil at various stages of pilot-plant refining and partial hydrogenation. J Am Oil Chem Soc 1978;55:616-618.

Elson CM, Ben EM, Ackman RG. Determination of heavy metals in a menhaden oil after refining and hydrogenation using several analytical methods. J Am Oil Chem Soc 1981;58: 1024-1026.

Ikekawa N, Matsui M, Yoshida T, Watanabe T. The composition of triglycerides and cholesteryl esters in some fish oils of brackish freshwater origin. Bull Jap Soc Sci Fish 1972;38: 1267-1274.

Ke PJ, Ackman RG, Linke BA. Autoxidation of polyunsaturated fatty compounds in mackerel oil: formation of 2,4,7-decatrienals. J Am Oil Chem Soc 1975;52:349-353.

Ratnayake WMN, Ackman RG. Fatty alcohols in capelin, herring and mackerel oils and muscle lipids. I. Fatty alcohol details linking dietary copepod fat with certain fish depot fats. Lipids 1979;14:795-803.

Ratnayake WMN, Olsson B, Ackman RG. Novel branched-chain fatty acids in certain fish oils. Lipids 1989;24:630-637.

Index